Practice Management
in Preventive Dentistry

Practice Management in Preventive Dentistry

A. Gary Dingerson, D.D.S.

Vancouver, Washington

Marilyn R. Dingerson, R.N., B.S.

Guest Lecturer,
Clark College Dental Hygiene Department
Vancouver, Washington

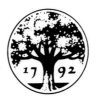

J. B. Lippincott Company

Philadelphia • Toronto

ISBN 0-397-50317-2

Library of Congress Catalog Card Number 73-8640

Printed in the United States of America

1 3 4 2

Library of Congress Cataloging in Publication Data

Dingerson, A   Gary
    Practice management in preventive dentistry.

    Bibliography: p.
        1. Dentistry—Practice.   2. Preventive
dentistry.   I. Dingerson, Marilyn R., joint author.
II. Title. [DNLM: 1. Practice management, Dental.
2. Preventive dentistry. WU113 D584 p 1973]
RK58.D5   617.6'01   73-8640
ISBN 0-397-50317-2

To those who
are dedicated
to the control
of Dental Disease

Preface

This book presents an organized approach to the control of dental disease and tells how prevention can be placed as the keystone in a dental practice. This approach, called *Preventive Dentistry*, holds to the premise that teeth are meant to last a lifetime and that the patient, through dental education and appreciation, can treat his own disease and bring it under control.

Dentistry is confronted with the most prevalent infection of mankind, dental caries and periodontal disease.[1] The Public Health Service estimates that 75 million adults have periodontal disease and that more than 20 million adults have lost their teeth because of this disease. They also state that four out of five children have gingivitis by the time they reach the age of 15. Yet, dental visits in a period of one year's time were calculated to be 3.6 per cent for the purpose of gum treatment.[2]

Dentistry, to be able to realistically solve the problems created by the magnitude of dental disease, should continue to increase the techniques to control disorders. The attempt is not to prevent dentistry, but to extend dental services through emphasis on prevention. This will enable the dental profession to take forward steps in providing the most complete and comprehensive dental care possible.

---

[1] National Institute of Dental Research: Research Explores Plaque. Bethesda, Md., National Institutes of Health, 1969, preface.

[2] National Institute of Dental Research: Research Explores Pyorrhea and Other Gum Diseases. rev. ed. Bethesda, Md., National Institutes of Health, revised 1972, pp. 3-5.

The ideas, methods, and data presented are intended to help put into the hands of the dentist and dental auxiliary the tools to conduct a disease control program and answer these and other questions:

1. Why a preventive practice?
2. What is a preventive practice?
3. What is the philosophy behind the preventive practice?
4. What are the facilities and equipment needed?
5. What is the role of the dental staff?
6. What are the tests and why do we need them?
7. How is a control program conducted?
8. When is a disease control program initiated within the treatment plan?
9. What should you say to patients?
10. How do patients respond to disease control?
11. How effective is a disease control program in controlling disease?
12. What are the rewards to the patient and to the staff?

Part I is devoted to giving dental personnel a perspective to create and carry out an effective program of dental education. Practice management has devoted much time and energy to developing a rapport with people so that what dentistry has had to offer would be more acceptable and more efficient. Now the attention of dentistry can be channeled to modify habits and behavioral patterns of dental patients for the purpose of directly combating dental disease. Each member of the dental health team will need to analyze his role in a patient education program, and suggestions are made to attain the objectives and goals set by the dentist and his staff.

Part II deals with the concepts and background information that are used as the basis for controlling dental disease, the nature of the disease processes, oral hygiene techniques, and nutrition as it is applied to dental disease. The removal of dental plaque and the measures for correcting faulty food selections and habits provide some very important answers and direction in solving the dentist's concern for better dental health. It applies to the patient's problems by providing solutions for achieving lasting and worthwhile results.

Part III gives a complete step-by-step procedure of how to attack dental decay and gum disease. It is not intended to imply that restorative procedures, equilibration of the teeth, scaling and polishing of the teeth, administration of fluorides, and other clinical measures are any less relevant today, but that an essential element of dental care is to give the patient the knowledge and the skills that he must have to obtain the benefits that can be achieved through control measures.

Changes are constantly occurring in the world we live in, and dentistry is no exception. Higher technology and scientific knowledge should be applied not only for the betterment of health, but also to increase the satisfaction of living. A breakaway from the past is in order, to establish an approach that will yield lasting results for the patient and provide the dental profession the rewards that come through service.

Each individual has different values, personality, past experiences, and life style. Hence, the approach to the control of dental disease will of necessity be different. The flexibility in the application of how to administer a control program will come through the thought and organization within each dental practice, and the program should be devised and arranged so that everyone concerned feels at ease and has the confidence that contributes to success. The techniques presented in this text should not be considered rigid in protocol but should serve as a stimulus to create and produce a workable preventive dental practice.

Shortcuts and deletions can deter and hamper combating the disease process, and any elimination of vital components, information, or techniques will contribute to less than satisfactory results. If the time, the interest, and the facts are given, then it is possible for every person to achieve lasting results and a healthy mouth.

It is hoped that this book will shorten the time necessary to incorporate control measures into a dental practice and that it may be helpful in strengthening an existing preventive practice by providing additional information.

We wish to express our appreciation to those who pioneered the knowledge and developed the educational skills that have placed preventive dentistry into the lives of people. We are indebted to those men and women who through their devotion to the profession have given their time and energy to look for better ways to practice and present dentistry.

The rationale, methods, and material furnished in this book were stimulated into being by the reports of Dr. C. C. Bass, Dr. Sumter Arnim, Dr. Arthur Alban, Dr. Robert Barkley, and the many others who have been acknowledged individually throughout the text. Through these people came the realization that there is a better answer to the age-old problem of dental decay and periodontal disease.

We extend a special thank you and sincere appreciation to Mrs. Ethel Hauser and Mrs. Barbara Holcomb, photographers, and to Mr. Gerald C. Scholle, medical illustrator, for the pictures and illustrations.

Our thanks to Mrs. Nancy Kennedy, C.D.A., for her assistance and contributions in establishing our preventive practice. We would particularly like to express our thanks to the J. B. Lippincott Company for recognizing the need for such a book.

A. GARY DINGERSON, D.D.S.
MARILYN R. DINGERSON, R.N., B.S.

Contents

A well-defined philosophy is necessary in adapting the concepts and techniques that interrelate to create a preventive dental practice.

Introduction

PREVENTIVE EQUATION OF DENTAL DISEASE

The disease process translated into the form of schematics or in terms of equations enables viewing the factors involved in a simplified straight-line relationship. By adding, subtracting, or altering the components, an effect can be exerted upon the final result. The initial illustrative equations for dental decay are:

FOOD (SUGAR) + BACTERIA = ACID
ACID + TOOTH = TOOTH DECAY

Other factors enter into these equations, but the chief concern in the past has been concentrated on the results produced by the interaction of the host with bacteria and their toxins. As the interest in controlling and preventing dental disease progresses, more attention is being diverted to modifying the variables by controlling the factors on the left side of the equations.

Caries has historically been treated by removal of the diseased tissue and repair or removal of the tooth. The changing of the environment of the tooth was previously attempted by admonishing the patient to brush after every meal and not to eat sweets. This method of control has been grossly inadequate. With the addition of fluorides to the community water supply and toothpastes and their use in topical applications to the teeth, it has been possible to modify and alter the severity of tooth decay.

The removal of bacteria from the tooth surfaces and underneath the gums by the once-a-day use of oral hygiene aids marked the advent of personal measures of disease control. The proper use of the toothbrush, dental floss, water irrigation, and periodontal aids, with the help of disclosing tablets or solutions, has appeal to the dentist and has advantages for people because of the improvement that can be experienced. It is the dental patient himself who ultimately assumes the responsibility to effect a change and control the factors involved. The disorganization of the dental plaque or dental microbiota focuses attention on the left side of the equation of dental disease and thus becomes a very important part of dentistry as a rationale for treatment.

A further shift to the left requires a concentrated effort to bring under control those food factors that are deleterious and promote dental disease. It is not enough to tell a patient to eliminate sweets; alternatives must be established. Nutrients that promote the prevention of dental disease and increase the resistance of the individual must be explored and recommended. The removal of the dental plaque is the first line of defense in preventive dentistry, but adding nutrition to the armamentarium makes control and prevention even more effective. Nutritional counseling permits treatment of the patient as a total person. It is not an easy task, but dentistry has accomplished many difficult tasks in the past.

PREVENTIVE COMPONENTS

The application of preventive measures requires changes in and additions to the dental practice. In structuring a preventive program, practice administration provides a method of operation so that more effort may be concentrated on the control and prevention of dental disease. Practice management is only a means to present a solid documented scientific program based on research. The methods used are designed to help the patient assimilate what dental science has to offer. By having an organized dental practice, dentistry is better equipped to apply what it has to offer so that results can be obtained, observed, and evaluated.

Prevention in dentistry means different things to the members in the dental health field, such as:

to restore a tooth
to scale and polish teeth
to instruct how to brush
to use systemic fluorides
to apply topical fluorides
to replace a tooth
to intercept malocclusions

Preventive dentistry also includes:

Plaque control:
Use of disclosants
Use of the phase microscope
Flossing
Brushing
Water irrigation
Periodontal aids and additional aids
Diet control
Nutritional counseling:
Food diary
Diet history
Computer analysis
Tests:
D-K test
Snyder's test for lactobacilli
Alkaline phosphatase test for streptococci (Stanton)

Acid phosphatase test for lactobacilli (Stanton)
15-Minute caries test (Rapp)
Lingual ascorbic acid test
Salivary and plaque tests

A host of other disciplines may also be included in the preventive concept, but the important point for the preventive dentist is that the etiological factors of dental disease be controlled.

THE APPEAL OF PREVENTIVE DENTISTRY

What is it that has stimulated so much interest in the dental health field to bring about renewed enthusiasm for oral hygiene procedures and ways of combating dental disease? It cannot be only the promise of successful results, but can it be the hope of achieving personal goals that have not been obtained previously by other methods? It is entirely possible that the dentist would like to eliminate the feeling of standing alone in the midst of fear, apprehension, decay, and gum disease and that he is searching for a means to alleviate the frustration that faces both the patient and the dentists because the contributing factors were previously left unchanged. Through education and communication the patient receives the message that action is required both by himself and by the dentist. When a total commitment is entered into by both parties, maximum satisfaction is achieved and the finest results in dental care can be accomplished.

Some major benefits for the dentist that are derived through a preventive practice:

1. A change in the patient's attitude toward dentistry.
2. The removal of the frustration of never-ending dental disease.
3. A greater acceptance of needed dental service.
4. An improvement in the health of the oral tissues, allowing better dentistry to be accomplished.
5. A greater appreciation of dentistry after it has been received.

DEVELOPING THE PHILOSOPHY

Each individual must seek for himself the answers that will formulate an image of what is needed, what can be accomplished, and how to proceed to arrive at the objectives and goals that are considered desirable.

Dr. Maxwell Maltz in his book, *Psycho-Cybernetics,* expresses the idea that conceived images provide a target that can be reached by making the necessary adjustments to home in on the objective just as an electronic missile adjusts to reach its destination.

In the past a model or a concept of preventive dentistry was lacking, making it difficult to comprehend or imagine practicing dentistry with the main purpose of controlling or preventing dental disease. One of the key figures in expressing new concepts and serving as a model for the preventive dentist is Dr. Robert Barkley. He has provided many guides by suggesting ideas and methods of application. He has shown how to realistically relate to people. Men such as Dr. C. C. Bass and Dr. Sumter Arnim have influenced Dr. Barkley's thinking and have given him guidance in developing this preventive consciousness.

The concepts and measures to provide prevention are becoming increasingly more available to the dental profession. With the rapidity and the number of views expressed, the overall continuity may appear clouded. This is a danger point because of the rationalization that may occur as a result of the confusion, the reluctance to change, or the feeling of inadequacy. This makes it even more important to establish a basic foundation of what prevention is and how it fits into a dental practice before an attempt is made to sort and sift the data and procedures into logical order. The ultimate success will be dependent upon how strong and how well a self-image is established of actually being a preventive dentist and visualizing what comprises one's ideals and dictates one's actions.

Postgraduate courses provide a source to stimulate and to furnish a new sense of direction for the staff and the dentist. The chief benefit of these seminars is that they relate clinical application and experiences for the dental profession to evaluate. However, in many instances participants in these lectures cannot fully realize the value of the material presented because of their lack of personal experiences within this field of prevention. The models and philosophies of others might indicate that certain ideologies are true, but it is only by experiencing them that they become reality.

The following questions may be of assistance in preparing a philosophy:

1. Do I believe in the preventive concept?
2. Do I believe the preventive concepts will work?
3. Do I really want to make the effort?
4. Can I provide a preventive program?
5. What are the goals of the dental health team?
6. What will the preventive program include? Plaque removal? Nutrition? Diet counseling? Use of fluorides?
7. Who will be in charge of the program?
8. When will it start?
9. When will the dentist and the staff have their own disease under control?
10. Will the teeth be cleaned professionally before or after the disease is controlled?
11. When will restorative treatment be initiated?
12. Will all patients be considered for control or just the ones selected?
13. What are the future plans of study for the dentist and his staff?

Further introspection after a program is instituted could include:

1. What is the difference between a preventive program and a preventive dentist practicing preventive dentistry?
2. Does the preventive concept include a comprehensive thorough diagnostic procedure as well as a complete disease control program?
3. If the patient decides not to proceed into prevention, what action serves the patient and dentistry best?

a. Does the dentist accommodate to fill the accepted needs of the patient?
b. Does the dentist serve only those patients who are willing to control and prevent their own disease?
4. What is the measure of success?

The final stage of developing a philosophy comes when it is placed on paper in written form. The dental auxiliary should be brought into the development of preventive concepts at the earliest opportunity. In this way each member of the dental staff will be able to contribute towards the development of the objectives and goals. It is through the services of the dental health team that a preventive program will be performed. A genuine devotion must be developed to serving people and to treating patients as total individuals. The impetus and final decisions will belong to the dentist, but it is the dental staff that makes it possible to provide preventive dentistry.

Time must be taken to plan so that a mental picture begins to develop of changes in the office layout, in systems, and in patient relations. It will not all come at once, but the growth that does occur will provide the stimulation that will carry through until the practice truly becomes preventive in scope. A definite plan is the surest and the most effective means of arriving at short-range goals and gives a more direct approach to achieving long-range goals.

PART I
The Personnel

1 | *Belief is turned into reality by taking the necessary steps to plan, design, create, and supervise a dental practice that is functional and structured to achieve the goals of prevention.*

The Role of the Dentist

APPLYING THE PHILOSOPHY

The advances in scientific knowledge, the comprehensive examination, the complete diagnosis, the disease control program, and the long-range planning will come to naught if a void is present between the patient and dentistry. Through a disease control program that "gives its all" to people, it is possible to bridge this gap. Dentistry is asking for greater responsibility from the patient in caring for himself, and this requires an even greater responsibility from dentistry in helping people help themselves. The motivation that comes to the patient will be brought about by his needs and promoted through the external stimulation of the dentist and his staff.

The effects of control should be evaluated by the patient in his own terms. If the dentist or the hygienist interjects his professional skill, for example, by scaling and polishing the teeth prior to the control program, it will not be possible for the patient to realize the full extent of what he can do for himself through the personal skills of oral hygiene. He has to do it for himself so that he can succeed and through this experience appreciate the contribution that the dental staff offers him.

The prevalence of dental disease is alarming. Many times symptoms do not indicate the extent or the true nature of the conditions that warrant control. Many people will show a greater than anticipated benefit from a

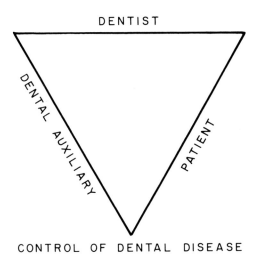

FIG. 1-1. Philosophy triangle.

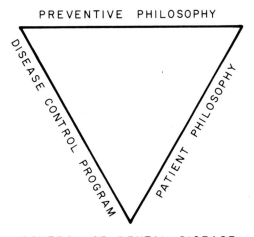

FIG. 1-2. Philosophy triangle.

3

disease control program. Any deviation from having a patient under control becomes second best.

Long-range follow-up should be available for and expected by both the patient and the dentist. The initial program should not block out further learning. People require reinforcement. They need to know if they are on the right track. If they are, they need to be congratulated, and if they are not, they can be further helped to gain self-motivation.

In order for the dentist to establish a preventive dental practice, he must make decisions and then delegate the responsibility of providing the program to the disease control therapist. He also delegates to the dental auxiliary, whether this be one or twenty, the role of reinforcing and assisting the patient, the dentist, and the disease control therapist in preventive procedures. The dentist finally delegates to the patient the controlling of his own disease.

A triangular diagram depicts the dentist, the dental staff, the patient, and their relationship to disease control (Fig. 1-1).

The control of dental disease occurs with the establishment of the preventive philosophy, the availability of the control program, and the development of the patient's philosophy (Fig. 1-2).

The many parts of the disease control program are conceived and systematically put together in a logical sequence. Modifications dictated by the patient's needs are made as required. The dentist must also reappraise what causes dental disease and give further consideration to his relationship with patients. Time is needed to think, to organize, and to investigate the ideas that appear to have merit. The ideal is difficult to attain, but movement in the direction towards prevention yields a condition much improved over what has gone before, nearer to the perfection that we seek in ourselves, and the improvement in the service we desire to give to others. The disease control program is not the goal. The goal is to control dental disease.

In addition to this, preventive dentistry provides the dentist with an opportunity for dynamic change. It is this concept that opens doors and provides an outlet for the previously learned basic sciences. This allows a direct application of the knowledge and the skills that the dentist possesses. This is of benefit to the patient because he is now being treated as a total individual. It changes the approach from simply going through the motions of brushing teeth or a discussion of food to a health service with real meaning and substance.

PLANNING THE FACILITIES

In the preventive dental practice the control program plays a major role in office management; therefore the area used to conduct the program should stand out as a place of importance within the office complex. The control room should indicate to the patient through its appearance that the dental health team considers this phase of dentistry of such value that an area was specifically designed to provide this service. The amount of space needed depends on the goals of the dentist and his staff and what the dentist intends to incorporate into the control program. Enough space should be made available so that both the patient and the disease control therapist will feel secure in their own territory (Fast).

The Need for Privacy

The single most important factor to be considered in selecting space for the control program is privacy for the patient and the disease control therapist. The patient and the control therapist must be able to work together without interruption or distraction from other patients or other members of the staff. This can be adequately handled by using a room that can be completely closed off. The disease control therapist is not just teaching the patient how to floss and brush his teeth; she is teaching him how to *treat* and control his disease. Patients do have emotional conflicts that require seclusion to be resolved. Conflicts can arise when the

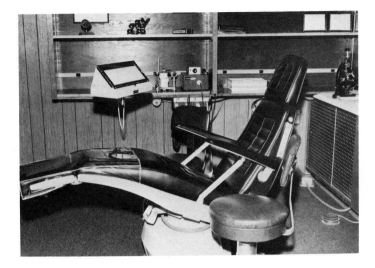

FIG. 1-3. A treatment operatory that also serves as a disease control operatory.

adult realizes that what he had previously been taught at both the parental and professional levels is not adequate. The child finds this new information is not what his teacher has taught him, and he feels as though he will get in trouble if he does not do what he has been previously taught to do, yet he wants to please his new friend, the disease control therapist. The patient with a denture may be especially sensitive and often requires additional considerations. To protect the patient's feelings, it is very important to provide privacy.

The Disease Control Operatory

In planning space for the control program two areas should be considered, one being the control room, which is used for the pro-

gram itself, and the second area, a disease control operatory (Fig. 1-3). The disease control operatory is primarily a treatment operatory that is used for Part A of control visit 1. It serves also as a back-up room for the program during busy hours or when several members of a family are seen at the same time.

In the disease control operatory, the sink is located in the cabinet behind the dental chair. The audiovisual equipment (Fig. 1-4) is located on a table across the room for viewing the filmstrip shown during the first part of disease control visit 1.

The Control Room

The space for the control room may be derived from an operatory not in use, a

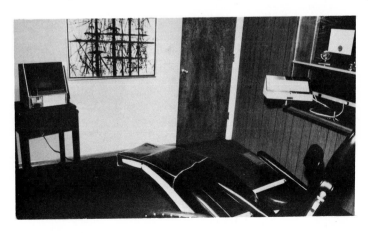

FIG. 1-4. Audiovisual equipment in a disease control operatory.

private office, or a large operatory that can be divided, redesigned, and equipped for control purposes. Reorganization of the office and the combining of activities may open up additional areas. (For example, move the facilities of a private office into a corner of the laboratory and redesign the private office into an examination and treatment operatory that also serves as a patient consultation room and a second control room.)

The dentist who is building or remodeling has the opportunity to design a room just for the purpose of "control." Regardless of the circumstances, the areas selected many times depend upon the imagination and determination of the staff.

Because of the personal nature of the control program, more lasting results are obtained when patients are treated on a one-to-one basis. Therefore, the room is not intended for use by more than several persons at one time. A suggested size would be that of an average dental operatory of 8

by 10 feet. It should be large enough to accommodate handicapped persons using crutches or wheelchairs. On occasion a mother may bring small children with her, and space is needed for a stroller or the toy box or whatever other means are devised to handle such situations.

The basic equipment for control rooms is a sink and mirror (Fig. 1-5). Two sinks, one for the patient and one for the control therapist, would be ideal. Hand washing by the control therapist is imperative; she may wash her hands up to four times during an appointment with a single patient. If the second sink is not available, the hands could be washed in a conveniently located clean-up area next to the control room.

The focal point of the room is where the action is, and that is the area in the immediate proximity of the patient's sink. The sink shown is built into a cabinet and placed slightly to one side of the center of the room (Fig. 1-6). With the sink in this position, the patient can view his entire surroundings; he

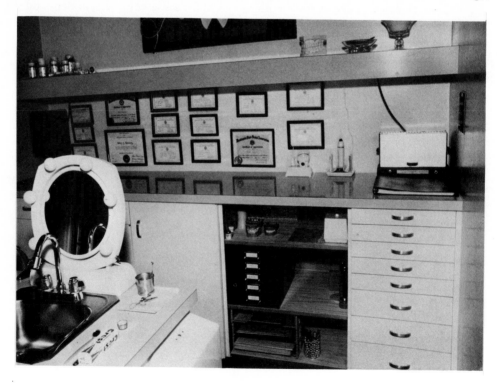

FIG. 1-5. A disease control room.

can see the wall hangings and equipment that are pertinent to the program. With this arrangement, the control therapist can sit or stand in front of the patient, allowing her to observe and instruct him. Knee space built into the front of the cabinet provides the patient more comfort in a sitting position. The inclusion of a bread board–style step allows small children to easily reach the sink.

Electrical outlets provided on the back of the cabinet supply the electricity for the oral hygiene aids that will be demonstrated and used. Doors on the back of the cabinet close off the area underneath the sink, making it possible to use this space for storage. Suitable lighting is obtained by using a makeup mirror that is attached to the back of the cabinet behind the faucets.

The counter space surrounding the sink provides space for a soap dispenser. On the right side of the sink, room is available for the patient's toothbrush, toothpaste, and mouth mirror, with the drinking cup, chest towel, and towel clips in the upper right corner.

The towel and paper cup dispensers are located on the right side of the cabinet with a closed waste receptacle close to the sink.

Dental stools are used by both the patient and the control therapist. These stools can readily be adjusted for all heights and sizes of patients.

A cabinet with counter space built along the back wall of the control room provides the shelves, drawers, and cupboards used for storage (Fig. 1-7). The counter is used during patient instruction and counseling. The area to the right of center could accommodate the second sink, which would be used by the control therapist. A series of

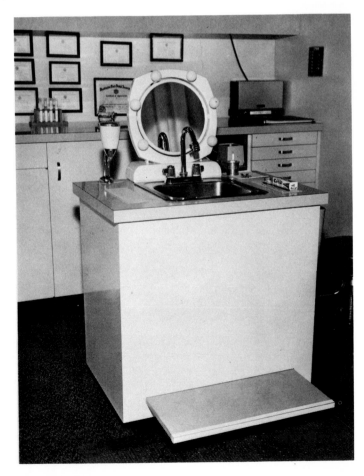

FIG. 1-6. The sink used for oral hygiene procedures.

drawers serve to hold the many small items such as the toothbrushes, floss, disclosing wafers, mouth mirrors, and other preventive supplies. In the section of the cabinet without doors, the shelves hold such items as the water sprays, test kits, flashlights, and demonstration models. These items that show add color and interest to the room. The more personal items such as the patient's toothbrush, diagnostic models, and chart are private and should be stored within the enclosed section of the cabinet. The shelf above the counter top holds books, various educational aids such as sugar jars for demonstration, and decorative plants or flower arrangements. A plug mold located under the shelf provides electricity for the incubator, x-ray view box, clock, and projector.

The room should be well lighted. This particular room has natural light provided by a skylight and indirect lighting located under the shelving above the counter top. If there are windows, they should be curtained. Light wall coverings will make the room seem larger. A selected color that complements the color scheme of the office can become officially designated as the control color. This color could be used in the covering of the cabinets, in the curtains, and in the carpeting as well as on the walls. The stationery as well as the instruments used within the control program can be color coded. Additional color and interest are derived from the bulletin board and wall charts that convey messages pertaining to the preventive program.

Carpeting is desirable but not essential. It does reduce the noise level, is easy to maintain, and makes the room appear pleasant and friendly. A piece of plastic floor runner placed immediately in front of the sink makes it easier to clean the spills that occur.

By providing facilities such as those described, the dental staff is telling the patient that there is far more to this program than just brushing the teeth. Having a room that is clean and professional will help to inform the patient of the staff's attitude towards what is being accomplished and convey to him that his privacy and dignity will be maintained.

EQUIPMENT

The major items of equipment are:
Phase Microscope — Model Mph-ZM
   Unitron Instrument Co.
   Microscope Sales Division
   66 Needham St.
   Newton Highlands, Mass. 02161
Projector and filmstrip or cassette for audiovisual presentation
   Dukane projector
   POH
   P.O. Box 45623
   Tulsa, Okla. 74145
      or
   Semantodontics
   P.O. Box 15668
   Phoenix, Ariz. 85018

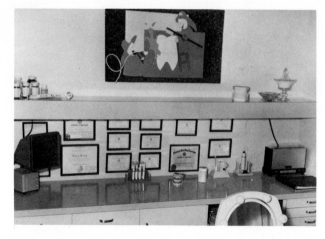

FIG. 1-7. Area for discussion and counseling.

Incubator (holds 21 test tubes)
   Thermolyne
   Dubuque, Iowa
X-ray view box for viewing x-ray films —
available from a dental supply house
Young's Caries Etiology Kit for testing
   Young Dental Manufacturing Co.
   2418 Northline Industrial Blvd.
   Maryland Heights, Mo. 63043

THE PREVENTIVE DENTAL STAFF

Prevention does not just happen, it is made to happen; it is people who make it happen for people. The initial motivation comes to the dental personnel through the dentist's desire to provide complete and effective dentistry for his patients. When the idea of prevention and control of dental disease catches hold of the staff, changes begin to occur. This can lead to even more cooperation among the members of the dental office. Helping people help themselves becomes more rewarding than just working for the public, for a dentist, or doing procedures to people. A greater respect is gained for the whole field of dentistry when the dental staff can improve its relationships with patients and can contribute a meaningful service.

It is through the dentist's leadership that the members of the staff function to establish this on-going commitment to dentistry. Because the greater responsibility (95 per cent) of the control program rests upon the actions and efforts of the dental auxiliary, their selection and development are of importance. The higher the plane that these individuals start from in terms of education, experience, abilities, and interests, the greater the potential for success. Those selected must be able to proceed logically from one step to the next without being inconsistent or irrelevant. They should be able to build on one idea after another. What is believed, personally practiced, and taught must be practical and capable of being carried out in daily situations; this can only be verified through the control of one's own disease.

The Obligation of the Staff

It becomes self-evident why the receptionist, assistants, hygienist, and the dentist should practice what they preach, but the laboratory man should not be left out of this discussion because the appliances that he constructs need to be adequately cleaned in the least amount of time and with the least number of cleaning aids. The embrasures, contour, and contact points take on more meaning when dental floss is to be used and the extent of bacterial involvement in the mouth is realized.

The control of disease in the mouths of the dental staff must be complete and not just token. The interpretation of what this means can be quite varied and will depend upon the definition of what contributes and constitutes health. It is possible to consider that health is achieved when in fact it is not. Health measures are not a one-time event but a constant striving for control and prevention. Health cannot be assumed; it must be constantly sought after. It is this search for health and the application of what is learned in the search that make up preventive dentistry.

It is not possible to conscientiously tell people about preventive dentistry when the instructor knows that his own teeth require restorations or the educator lacks experience.

The Disease Control Therapist

The preventive nurse, disease control therapist, or whatever name given, may be a dental hygienist, a certified dental assistant, a registered nurse, or a schoolteacher. Such a person serving in this capacity would already have specialized training that would be helpful in conducting a program of this type. However, it is more than likely that the person delegated will be untrained in the field of dentistry or the related sciences or both. Since the preventive practice is dependent upon the disease control therapist, the selection should be made carefully. The attributes of an individual are not easily listed in systematic fashion, but each person has characteristics and traits that can be molded and developed to serve himself and others satisfactorily.

Personal qualities can best be viewed in light of the duties that are necessary appointment after appointment, day after day. The person selected must be intelligent and able to understand the processes of dental disease and how they are related to dental treatment. The abilities of the individual should include the capacity to select materials and techniques that will inform and motivate the patient, and then the individual must be able to relate this information to the many different types of personalities. The control therapist will continually be making emotional adjustments to meet needs as they arise at any given moment. The person selected must be emotionally stable within herself.

The control therapist must have a strong positive mental attitude in contrast to someone who cannot see the "silver lining." The control therapist will at times be dealing with negative problems and negative people, and each situation must be viewed optimistically and with the knowledge that positive results can and will be achieved. This confident and optimistic attitude enables her to handle situations to a successful outcome. It is the enthusiasm radiated by the control therapist that will help convince the patient that he should make the effort to change his habits and take over the responsibility of caring for himself.

The techniques and procedures of the control program may be routine, but the patients are not, and this requires patience and understanding. People come in all ages, all types of personalities, and with all degrees of oral disease. All have their own peculiarities. Adequate manipulation of the fingers in handling the floss may be difficult for some patients, and, in order to accomplish the art, the learner needs the support of a patient, understanding, and competent teacher. The problems that arise must be solved with ease and without frustration or irritation. The patient is the concern—not the feelings, need, or time schedule of the

control therapist. Most important, there must be respect for each person and a sincere attempt at understanding the feelings and motives of people. It will be her task to teach all she knows about the disease in such a way that the patient will most likely be motivated to make it his to use for the remainder of his life.

It is to the dentist's advantage that the control therapist has full or at least partial dentition in optimum condition, and that she be in good physical health. As soon as she becomes the control therapist she is a living example of what the dentist expects of his patients. If her experience approximates that which the patient will undergo, then she will be able to realize the transformation that occurs and appreciate what a really clean mouth feels like. She can more effectively teach patients after overcoming difficulties that she may have had in changing her own habits. In this way, she will be able to say to patients that she has not missed flossing her teeth since the day she started, which may be 1 month or 4 years, and she will know what it is to follow the basic four food groups, eliminate sugar, and feel the effect of adequate nutrition.

The dentist gives to the control therapist the understanding that the control program is hers to succeed. The goals of the program are her goals also. Although directed by the dentist or the dental hygienist, it is primarily her responsibility, and she should be able to implement the program in such ways as she sees fit. As she works with patients, new and better ways of doing things will be learned. By continually studying and selecting new material and information as it becomes available through research, and deleting from the program the material that becomes outdated and incorrect, the program can be kept current and interest kept alive.

If untrained in dentistry, she will need a great deal of assistance from the other members of the dental health team. Regardless of her background, she will need time to think, to plan, and to study. It will be through her that a program is developed, and it would seem unwise to give a certain trial period to learn or develop it. This probationary approach does not provide security for the newly employed person and, in fact, gives the suggestion of failure. Unsatisfactory personnel should be dismissed early in employment because the longer dismissal is delayed the more difficult it becomes. The attitude, enthusiasm, and motivation towards the preventive concept are the important factors, and these are evident and show signs of maturing within the first week of employment.

Credit needs to be given to the control therapist from the members of the dental team, including the dentist. The results that are achieved will bring justification for such praise, but these facts must be communicated. The zeal and enthusiasm, some of the essentials for a successful preventive practice, come as a result of bringing mouths under control, improving patient relationships, furthering the patient's understanding of dentistry, and then receiving the recognition that it was made possible through the efforts of the control therapist.

Utilizing the Dental Auxiliary

The dentist derives a tremendous amount of encouragement and stimulation in developing a preventive program from the members of his own staff. Another preventive practice can serve as a model, but it is the members of the staff who must visualize and function to initiate this type of dental service. By the staff's working together, ideas emerge that will be far more relevant and adaptable than is possible with each member working separately.

Staff meetings provide an occasion where the basic elements are discussed and the initial training occurs. It is in these sessions that individual contributions will produce the parts of the total structure to make it work. A feeling of accomplishment and personal satisfaction is obtained when results are reached, and a closer working relationship is formed by practicing together as a team. The staff meetings are not sessions to delegate duties but are for the purpose of idea development and problem solving. The goals of these meetings will change in character as the goals and the objectives are met. Projects will have to be delegated by the dentist, but it is preferable that the personnel have their duties come to them as a natural outgrowth of what is needed. With this approach, motivation will be present to provide the maximum effort for the successful completion of the project. With each individual accepting responsibility for specific tasks, the overall load will be lessened. When each member is in tune with what is planned and what others are accomplishing, there is less opportunity for omissions and overlapping of tasks. Topics for these meetings will be selected by the dentist, but he may choose to have a staff member initiate and lead the discussions. A positive attitude should be maintained, and the staff meetings should not be allowed to become negative. The dentist should listen and not discourage the member of the staff who questions the approaches to be taken or who is critical of steps that are considered. This person provides a balance that helps to illustrate points that do require more research, more effort, and more consideration. All members of the staff should appreciate the importance and the need for a person who is sincerely concerned and can view all the factors involved. However, a totally negative attitude can be destructive. If the dentist had a negative attitude, the disease control program would of course not have been considered. If a negative attitude is present in one member, the program can be threatened, and it will be a definite detriment to the other members of the staff.

The program for staff meetings will include the development of the preventive philosophy for the dental office and consideration of the best means of implementing this philosophy into the dental practice. Postgraduate courses provide motivational stimuli and should be attended by all members of the office. The staff meeting following such seminars are used to evaluate the information received and to consider its application within the existing program. Dental literature provides a similar opportunity, and all members should be encouraged to read selected articles considered by the dentist or other staff members to be applicable to the preventive practice. After each staff member has read the material, it is initialed and passed on to the next person. Other areas to be considered in the staff meetings may be the development of the control program, ordering supplies, training of auxiliary, improving existing facilities, appointment and traffic control. Other discussions can be held concerning job description, chair-side techniques, patient relations, communications, diet, and nutrition.

The dentist should take a moment to enjoy this stimulation of a practice that is blossoming into the field of prevention. It is a very exciting time.

The personnel should develop flexibility and become knowledgeable in the roles of the other staff members so that they may be able to assist or replace each other in times of need. This refers to daily need and not specifically during times of illness or emergencies. Patients are people, and people and their schedules are not routine. There are many times when it would seem that there is not sufficient staff to handle the control program. It is at this time that assistance must come from other personnel, whether receptionist, dental hygienist, another assistant, or a bookkeeper. With this type of team work, true appreciation, understanding, and respect will radiate into the entire office, and it will help to develop a real sense of loyalty to one another.

For stability, continuity, and success of the program, one person should be considered in charge of the control program. She should be trained as the control therapist and be considered the key member in the preventive team that provides the control program for patients. The work of the control therapist is not piecework, and it should not be viewed as a task where remuneration is received for each service. At least one other member of the staff should be trained as the control therapist so that she may assist during extremely busy hours and act as relief during the regular therapist's absence.

Where does the control therapist come from? The dental office can, of course, hire a person to be the control therapist. In some instances the wife of the dentist may volunteer to accept the position. This may be especially true if she is an experienced dental assistant, hygienist, registered nurse, or a teacher. Regardless of her training and background, it is a fortunate dentist who has the assistance of his wife because of the many additional hours of planning and developing the program that in all probability she will provide. If an assistant is selected from the existing staff, she will already have a background in dentistry and will more easily be able to adjust to this new role. The dentist will also know her emotional and physical capabilities, which will be a help in this decision. Assignment of duties may take the form of:

An office with two auxiliaries: One auxiliary would serve as an assistant-receptionist, the second serving as the control therapist. The disease control therapist could assist with the telephone and patient correspondence and help the assistant-receptionist in a limited capacity.

An office with three auxiliaries: One auxiliary would serve as the receptionist, the second auxiliary would serve as assistant to the dentist, and the third auxiliary would be the control therapist.

Another possibility would be to hire a person in addition to other personnel who could be trained in the duties of the assistant to serve during peak hours. This would free an assistant for preventive appointments during this period.

PRESENTING THE NEED

The exchange of amenities that occur between the patient and the dental office staff develops rapport. The dentist through his technical training is able to demonstrate directly, in the patient's mouth, and indirectly, by the use of x-ray films, diagnostic models, tests, microscopic examination, and verbal communications, the condition that exists. Pathological changes can be shown from the smallest detail, such as the bacteria in the microscope, to bleeding of the gums and gross loss of bone as well as the extent of dental decay that has destroyed the tooth structure. And yet, in spite of all that can be said and done by the dentist, what really matters is the patient's reaction. What has not changed are the patient's past experiences and his values.

It is the dentist's responsibility to examine and diagnose, to establish a treatment plan, and to inform the patient of his dental needs as well as what he may expect in the future if certain courses are followed. The awareness of the dentist becomes even more acute when it is found that steps can be taken to correct the conditions concerning periodontal disease and the factors that cause dental decay. If the patient is not allowed to go through the same process of evaluation and if he is not helped to develop a philosophy towards prevention, then a situation arises that leads to his inability to realize the need for change. It may be that part of the fear of dentistry can be attributed to the fear the patient has of losing control over a situation that is dominated by the dentist in ascertaining what needs to be corrected and how it should be accomplished. Dentistry is not a game of choice, but there is a choice of taking steps to correct inadequate conditions. Preventive education is that extra step needed to express the facts and make possible full acceptance by the patient.

The formal dental examination as outlined in Chapter 7 provides a logical and controlled entrance of the patient into a disease control program. Specific needs should be satisfied before the examination. It is better to treat emergency patients (toothache, broken tooth, or repair of a broken partial denture) and advise them of their need for an examination procedure than to interject the need for a disease control program. If the emergency involves a highly demon-strable periodontal disease and the patient requests to have his teeth cleaned, then control of disease could profitably be instituted prior to the examination. Dental education is greatly reduced when the short-term approach of repair or treatment is utilized as the only means of service; learning will not take place if high-priority patient needs are left unfulfilled. Variations in the order of treatment depend upon the needs of the patient, and the order to be followed depends on the judgment of the dentist.

The dentist should forget that he has a disease control program and remember that dentistry consists of finding a solution to the patient's problems, not of creating a new one. Focusing attention on the control program should be avoided in order to prevent blocking of future avenues of learning in this field and too much emphasis on the program at the expense of the needs of the patient. Statements should be designed so as to not progress into questions that become more involved and end in confusion because of lack of organization of thought by the dentist and inadequate preparation of the patient to comprehend the answers. There is plenty of opportunity for the dentist to tell all he knows and to go further into explanations within the disease control program itself. This will take practice; at first there will be slips, but success will eventually come. It is the only way to bring the patient into the program fresh and eager to learn. It is within the program that the patient is ready for information that falls in correct and logical sequence, and the patient is geared to skill development and becoming involved.

Presenting the need does not occur at one point in time called the consultation appointment. It occurs between the initial contact of the patient with the dental office and the time he says, "Yes, I wish to do what is necessary to correct the situation and control my disease."

Arriving at an Understanding

The dental examination ceases to be solely a means of discovering symptoms but becomes a time when the dentist and the patient come together to learn about each other and to find the extent to which dental health can be promoted both now and in the future. The dentist communicates to the patient possible solutions to problems in such a manner as to provide hope rather than despair. The whole process proceeds without recrimination or criticism of what brought about the destruction, and the patient is led to the realization that what has occurred is a disease, the most prevalent infection of mankind.

It takes two people to communicate, and time is necessary to produce a relationship that yields more than just a transient response. In order to be effective, the dentist and his staff must *listen* and establish a rapport that is sympathetic and understanding. The patient is made ready to listen by reducing his inner fears and prejudices that block out any exchange of information. The first step is to accept people as they are with their unique personalities and their own beliefs and wishes for themselves.

A schematic of the route that a patient may follow through a dental practice is shown in Figure 1-8.

The dental examination provides the key to getting to know the patient and establishing a personal relationship with the goal of better dental health. The patient is not impressed with what we know; he is impressed by what we know about him. People do not fit into fixed patterns; their reactions are unpredictable. Their needs are at times hard to determine but evident if we but look.

The dentist's methods of practice administration should allow the patient to express *his* philosophy and provide freedom of expression. The dentist's procedures should enable him to be flexible and allow him to search for the proper perspective so that each patient's personality, wants, and needs can be properly determined. The dental examination is the listening device, not merely a platform for the motivation and the changing of the patient's behavior. It is hoped that through the dental examination people will come to understand and appreciate what dentistry has to offer, but the dentist should come away from the examination believing that he too has learned by knowing the patient better both clinically and personally.

An Overall View of the Three-Phase Examination

Phase I consists of establishing a good emotional atmosphere. The attitude of the dentist can be expressed to the patient and the patient's past dental experiences explored. The patient's interest and reactions as related to dentistry are discussed in order to reveal what feelings are present towards dental treatment and his expectations for treatment. This provides a basis for further communication. Questions are asked, and the dentist listens to hear the patient express his own specific needs.

Communication occurs when the patient expresses himself fully. Conversation should not consist of trying to please the dentist or telling the dentist what he wants

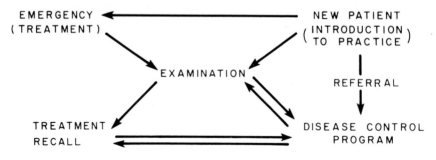

FIG. 1-8. Treatment routes in the preventive dental practice.

to hear but should be a true expression of what is on the patient's mind.

The second step, or Phase II, in the examination uses the tools of diagnosis — study models and x-ray and visual examinations. The demonstration and conversation are frank, honest, matter-of-fact, in depth, and in terms that the patient can understand and appreciate. The patient actually experiences seeing the dentist at work, learning and discovering what he is like as a person.

The examination begins the asking of questions and the finding of answers. At this time it is established whether dental disease is present and, if it is, that the patient realizes it is happening to him. The prospect of dental disease is faced by each of us for we do not live in a sterile world. The extent of symptoms varies. If gross symptoms are present, measures are taken to control the disease. Otherwise these same measures are instituted to prevent disease.

It is towards this realization in the dental examination that the dental patient is aligned with a philosophy that leads to the acceptance of the preventive method of dental care. The patient's awareness of his own personal involvement is increased. He may know that he has cavities or bleeding gums, but in all probability he does not consider it a disease or an infection. From this recognition comes the decision to do something about it. He is not informed of the what and the how this is done; that is left until the disease control program.

The third step is for the dentist to express in written form the evaluation, diagnosis, treatment plan, and prognosis. The emphasis is on thoroughness, clearness, and developing a plan that meets the needs of the patient as well as sets a course for the patient to follow. Decisions have been made by the dentist, but the patient has been exposed to the conditions that brought about these decisions in Phase II of the examination.

It is the conviction and the knowledge of the dentist that help the patient catch hold of the concepts and the importance of combating dental disease. The patient has to under-

stand the new roles of each of the participants, the dentist, the dental staff, and himself, so that he can easily fit into and adjust to becoming involved and a contributing member. The sequence of events becomes more effective when it satisfies a need and the patient is able to receive information and then directly apply and develop a personal skill. The true beginning occurs when the patient starts to think in terms other than just what conditions exist and takes action to modify the factors that contribute to the problem.

It may not always be possible for the dentist to reach his goal and satisfy his philosophy for every dental patient. The patient may have other needs of greater importance to him than his dental needs. What is achieved is a clear understanding of the extent of cooperation that can be expected. By being able to better understand people and having a clearer conception of how dental disease can be conquered, it is possible to more fully cope and master the many different situations that arise.

Inaugurating the Program

The practice of preventive dentistry begins with basic concepts and proceeds with the development of goals and procedures. As these are reached, new ones are set. The practice of today is just an extension of yesterday's methods and techniques. What is added is built upon the foundations from the past. A start has to be made or the plans for the future will never come true.

Basically we are dealing in two areas, oral hygiene and nutrition. They become more complex as we go deeper into the understanding of their whys and wherefores. After a thorough study and evaluation of all factors it comes back full cycle that the important area of consideration in this field is the direct application of oral hygiene and nutrition. When this phase of dentistry is attended to, other forms of treatment can be accomplished with more confidence and pride. The patient is making his contribution and learning about himself. A major part of the disease control program is purely motivational to reach this goal of patient commitment.

As the dental office begins its program, the members of the staff may be relying upon the experience of those who have gone before. To build confidence, they should begin with the patient who knows that he has bleeding gums and does not need a dentist to tell him so. Such patients are receptive, and the results in a very short time are comparable to a miracle. From then on the staff will know that the program is acceptable and workable.

Only by doing and by seeing the results will the dental staff gain the knowledge that reinforces the effort and helps them to continue on the path of prevention. As with everything, there will be moments of discouragement, but it will be at these same moments that a patient will present himself in such need, or results are obtained that are so gratifying, that the staff members wonder why they ever doubted.

The control therapist provides the link between dental science and the application of what controls dental disease. She is the key figure in translating dental education into positive action for the benefit of the dental patient.

The Role of the Disease Control Therapist

THE CHALLENGE

The personal service that is to be provided can only successfully be given by one who is positive, patient, understanding, and sensitive to people and their needs. The basic means of applying disease control is through verbal and nonverbal communication between the patient and the educator. The resulting effects of the program on the patient and the relationships that are formed will be both direct and indirect, tangible and intangible. The control therapist must handle the control program with conscientious care. She must have the capacity to develop.

The people who will be counseled within a general dental practice are of all ages with varying degrees of oral disease, personal frustrations, and problems. There is a vast opportunity to learn and grow from the experiences of working with this great variety of people. The personal exchanges that take place should occur in a relaxed and enjoyable atmosphere so that the patient and the control therapist can relate to each other to find solutions to the problems at hand.

The first priority for the control therapist is to have a complete understanding of what preventive dentistry means and to apply its principles to the care of her own mouth. It cannot be done in token only; it *must* be believed and practiced.

The ultimate success of the control therapist depends upon her willingness to give of herself to help other people. This is a prime factor in the motivation of herself as well as in the influence that she will have on the patient. This is reflected in the ability to listen and to understand what the patient is saying and to bring into perspective the subject matter that will be meaningful to the individual.

The Responsibilities

In meeting this challenge of preventive dentistry, the responsibility of the control therapist as outlined in this text will be to instruct the patient in oral hygiene techniques (Chapter 5), to perform salivary testing (Chapter 4), and to counsel in nutrition (Chapter 6). The dentist, through the diagnosis, informs the patient of the extent of his disease and helps to develop the awareness that he can take steps to control it (Chapter 7). It is not the task of the control therapist to motivate the patient, but it is her assignment to assist the patient in *motivating himself.* Patient motivation results from the changes that he personally experiences. It is furthered through the instruction he receives concerning the conditions that exist in his mouth and what can be done to restore and rehabilitate this destruction and, finally, by becoming knowledgeable concerning his future dental care.

It becomes an overall understanding by the patient of his dental needs and an appreciation of dentistry through education.

Planning the Program

Dental education takes place far more effectively within the framework of the control program. Here the patient is willing to give the time to learn "why it needs to be treated" in contrast to the "how-long-is-it-going-to-take?" attitude encountered in the treatment situation. The examination and treatment appointments are not conducive to the learning process because the tensions that are associated with general dentistry are too high.

The Goals. The short- and long-range goals of the control program should be considered by the dentist and the control therapist as they prepare the material and determine the number and arrangement of appointments.

Suggested short-range goals:

1. That the patient will learn to adequately clean his teeth.
2. That the patient will analyze his food selections and eating habits and that he will correct and change them if necessary to help insure good dental health.
3. That the patient will become stimulated, enthusiastic, and motivated to return for each subsequent appointment.

Suggested long-range goals:

1. That the patient will continue to establish the habit of adequately cleaning his teeth after he has completed the specified number of appointments and that he realizes he has not just gone through a program, but that he is on a program that will continue throughout his lifetime.
2. That the patient will incorporate into his life style the selection of food that will increase those nutrients that will allow him to be more physically fit and mentally alert.
3. That the patient will accept the responsibility to continue to keep his mouth free of dental disease.

The Number and Length of Appointments. Enough time must be allowed to achieve the goals of the program. The number of appointments and the time-space relationship between visits are determined by that which is needed to treat the disease and alter the habit patterns. The length of each appointment is determined by the amount of educational material to be presented and the capacity of the patient to receive.

Multiple appointments close together followed by several spaced at intervals appear to be the most effective. Five visits as close together as possible during a 7- to 10-day period allow the patient to learn the techniques and help him to establish the habit of flossing daily. The single most important motivational factor is the feel that the patient experiences as the mouth changes from one that is dirty to one that is clean. This change occurs during the first several days. Appointments close together insure the proper cleaning so that this change does occur and is recognized by the patient. An appointment one week following the initial five visits provides further assistance and allows the patient to evaluate his progress after he has practiced the skills alone.

Another appointment is scheduled in 1 month. By this time the patient has found and developed the most comfortable method of handling floss. Often the patient will have modified the brushing technique, which is acceptable providing he continues the sulcular brushing and adequately removes the plaque. This appointment also enables the control therapist to evaluate the effectiveness of the control program. The last appointment in the series of eight is held 2 months from the previous appointment. At this visit the patient reaffirms his goals to control his disease. During the interval, the patient may have lapsed into old habits; the techniques may have slipped and become inadequate, resulting in symptoms of sore and bleeding gums. If this occurs, the patient has learned how easy it is for the disease to return. He knows how to correct it; he has learned by trial and error. He must decide for himself if he wants a mouth free of disease or if he wants an unhealthy mouth that can threaten his total being.

The Content of the Program. To best achieve the goals of the program the patient should clean his teeth during each control appointment under the supervision and the encouragement of the control therapist. Many obstacles can deter the patient during the learning process. The patient with tender and bleeding gums needs the daily support of the control therapist in order to continue. If he is left to do it alone at home, it may not be done because he thinks the gums are too sore. The child needs the attention daily not only to learn the technique but also as a reminder not to forget to do it.

Some patients can and will master the skills very rapidly, but they have not developed the habit. To change habits they must know why it is necessary in their own mouths. The patient must realize that his teeth are *his*, that they are a part of him, and that it is up to *him*, not the dentist, to prevent disease. He must know the how, why, what, and when dental disease can and does take place in his mouth, in his spouse's mouth, in his children's mouths, and even in the mouths of his friends and relatives. For further patient understanding and motivation, informative material should be incorporated into the program that is personalized and relates directly to him and his family. The material and information used within the control program reflect the philosophy of the dental office. The dentist may wish to outline the material to be incorporated into the program. From there, the control therapist can plan it in logical sequence and write it down. Regardless of the past experience or training that the control therapist brings to the control program, there are several things to keep in mind:

1. What would I like to know about my teeth if I knew nothing at all?
2. What is it in the information, aids, or presentation that would keep me interested so that I would eagerly return for each of the scheduled appointments?

The dental information that is added at each appointment serves many functions, some of which are:

For the patient:

1. It allows the patient an opportunity to relax after completing the task of flossing and brushing the teeth.
2. It exposes the patient to valuable information concerning his teeth that in the past he felt was not his to know.
3. It tells the patient why this must be done in his mouth to save and prevent further destruction of his teeth and surrounding bone structure.
4. It gives the patient an opportunity to think and learn about his dental conditions and ask questions concerning them.
5. It prepares the patient for future dental treatment.
6. It stimulates the patient and encourages him to return for each of the scheduled appointments.
7. It tells the patient that the dental health team is providing this program because the members care for him as a person and not just for monetary reasons.
8. It assists him to change his deleterious habits to more helpful ones.

For the control therapist:

1. The discussion that occurs between the patient and the control therapist establishes invaluable rapport.
2. The discussions inform the control therapist what the patient knows about his teeth, what he considers to be important, and what he intends to do about it. This information is essential if she is to present a personalized program to the patient that will result in altering his habits. The indirect method of obtaining information is more discreet and considerate and often leads to obtaining more information and better understanding.

To conduct the program the control therapist should have, in addition to knowing the oral hygiene techniques, a knowledge of basic dental science, an understanding of bacteriology, diet and nutrition, and human relations. There should be a review of the major research that provides the foundation for the control of dental disease as we know it today. This information provides the control therapist with an inner sense of security and self-assurance that comes through total comprehension of the subject. It also serves as a source to draw upon to answer the questions asked by the patients. The answers need not be technical because this is not what the patient needs or desires, but the information given should be knowledgeable and accurate. The answers given serve to allay fears, help solve problems, and assist the patient in deciding the course of future dental treatment. Frequently it plants a new seed of interest that may alter or change the lives of people.

If a question is asked that cannot be answered, the patient should be assured that an attempt will be made to find the answer for him by the next visit. It is not possible to know all the answers, nor is it wise to consider that all the answers are known. What is felt by the patient is the positive attitude of the control therapist, and he is more impressed with this than with a quick answer for every question.

The control therapist, regardless of her previous experience, must remember as she works with the patient that she is the teacher, that the program is excellent, and that she has been adequately trained for this position.

Assembling the Information

As data are accumulated, a file should be started listing the subject and the source. This is invaluable for future reference.

A second file is also suggested for the purpose of collecting information coming through the mail. It can be separated according to company or product, or both, and subject matter. What is not needed today may be useful tomorrow.

Specific areas of learning for the control therapist:

Basic Dental Science

Sources: Dental assistant textbooks, dental books, the dentist, and the dental hygienist

Information to review:
  Structures of the oral cavity
    Anatomy of the mouth
    Anatomy of the tooth
    Primary teeth and their relationship to permanent teeth
  Oral pathology
    Caries
    Pulpitis
    Periapical abscess
    Gingivitis
    Periodontitis
  Diagnostic tools
    X-ray examination
      Types: Bite-wing, apical
      Value: Development and placement of teeth
        Caries determination
        Periodontal involvement—extent of bone loss
  Vitalometer
  Transillumination
  Treatment
    Dental materials
      Gold
      Amalgam
      Plastics
    Types of restorations
      Three-quarters and full crown
      Porcelain and porcelain to gold
      Surface restorations—mesial, distal, occlusal, lingual, buccal
    Permanent and removable appliances
      Bridges
      Partials
    Pulpotomies
    Endodontia
    Extractions
    Fluoride
      The mechanism of how it works
      Who should receive it
      Availability—tablets, drops, toothpaste, topical application, water supply
      How often it should be used

Etiology of Dental Disease (Chapter 4)

Sources: Dental assistant textbooks, dental reference books, scientific papers selected by the dentist

Microbiology

Bacteriology

Nutrition (Chapter 6)

Sources: Dental assistant books, books on nutrition and the teaching of nutrition, articles by the National Dairy Council

Understanding People

Sources: Dental assistant books, psychology books written for teachers and nurses, child development books and pamphlets, books on communicating with people

Specific References for

Background Information

Dental Disease (sources): Research articles by Dr. Sumter Arnim, available through Dr. M. Wheatcroft, Professor of Pathology, The University of Texas at Houston, Dental Branch. Books— Amenta and Brackett; Barkley; International Conference on Dental Plaque (see Bibliography)

Nutrition (sources): Books and articles— Clark, Cheraskin, and Ringsdorf; Eat to Live; Indications of nature of food relationships in caries; National Research Council—Food and Nutrition Board; Nizel 1972 (see Bibliography)

Patient Relations (sources): Berne; Fast; Ginott; Maltz; Weiss and Swearingen (see Bibliography)

Preparing the Visual Aid

A visual aid assists the control therapist in teaching the patient. It helps the patient to understand that which is being taught. In selecting visual aids for the control program, two objectives should be continually kept in mind:

1. Does the visual aid give authority to the program?

2. Can the information presented in the visual aid be related to the mouth of the patient or his family or his friends?

The visual aid must be selected with extreme care. The picture, model, or filmstrip must be consistent with the philosophy of the control program. It cannot say one thing and the dentist and the control therapist say another.

The visual aids will vary with each control program because they reflect the need of the program and the personality of the control therapist. They should be planned as an integral part of the appointments and follow in logical sequence in order to accomplish the purpose for which they are intended. For example, the patient should not view a film prior to an appointment session if he will not understand or appreciate its message.

Take-home material can be considered a visual aid and must be selected with the same care. The amount of material should be minimal in number and high in quality. When a patient responds to receiving a pamphlet by saying, "Oh Good," or if he grabs it from the control therapist, then this is what the patient needs and desires.

General information for the patient to take home can include:

1. Pamphlet describing the control program. (This tells the patient what it is all about.)

2. Pamphlet illustrating the oral hygiene techniques. (This tells the patient how to do it.)

3. Pamphlet informing what has been accomplished. (This tells the patient the results that are obtainable.)

The printed take-home material is given the patient because the control therapist believes that he will benefit from its information and because people like to take things home, especially if they are given to them. All the information and "goodies" should not be given at one time. The patient will not read a total package of material, nor is he prepared to understand it. To keep the interest alive and anticipation high, information should be distributed at appropriate places throughout the eight control visits. Printed materal should be reviewed with the patient so that he understands the information. He should not be depended upon to read and study it at a later time. If the information is of such importance that it belongs in the organized control program, then it is equally important that the patient understand it during the scheduled appointment.

Creating the Records

It is essential that a chart be prepared to record the response of the patient to treatment. It is suggested that abbreviations not be used in the charting. Use of abbreviations may shorten the charting time, but only the personnel who made the abbreviations will know what they mean.

The chart can be in the form of a check list (Chapter 8). It is best not to alter the basic content of the material presented at each visit, but instead to adapt it to each individual patient in order to meet his needs. The check list prevents the omission of vital information.

Additional records will be discussed in the sections dealing with their use.

A system grading the ability to clean teeth and subsequently control disease is not used in the control program of this text. These systems can be a degrading factor in patient relationships if not handled properly. The ability involved in adequately cleaning the teeth is highly individualized, and some patients require months or even years to acquire the skill. A grading system may be desirable for academic or research purposes, but the compliments and the recognition of patient progress towards a goal are what achieve results.

RELATING TO PEOPLE

Success depends on the ability of the patient to make behavioral changes in the manner in which he cleans his teeth and in the methods by which he sustains life through the foods he eats.

One of the basic needs of all persons is to be an adequate individual. An individual's self-respect is preserved by what others give to him in the way of recognition and a sense of worth. A person never outgrows the need for preservation of self-esteem, and if this is maintained, positive results will be enhanced. The concept of self occurs in how a person sees himself, how he would like others to see him, and how he sees other people. A healthy person will think well of himself by having positive experiences, by being able to accept and handle negative facts, by being able to identify with people, and by being understanding and able to give of himself. A mature person can face the truth of a situation; he can accept responsibility for himself and others and act rightly. He treats people as people rather than as objects, its, or things.

All persons have attitudes. Attitudes are a system of negative and positive, pro and con emotional feelings. They determine how we see ourselves, what we hear, how we think, and what we do. They are shaped by the information that the person is exposed to, providing it meets his needs. Attitudes are related to the group with whom the person affiliates and also reflect his personality.

In order for behavior to be changed, attitude must first be changed, and this is fostered through information. What is given must be worthwhile and of value to the patient, and it must meet his needs. The more intelligent the person, the more able he is to handle the negative data that are involved because of the defense mechanisms he has built up. Tension, conflict, and frustrations occur and are present during change. The control therapist must inform the patient through communications that she will help him, that he is safe and secure, that his dignity will be preserved, and that he will not be hurt "by me." Through this security the patient can receive negative data and effectively learn and change his behavioral habits.

The control therapist has her program material well planned and organized. She does not have a speech prepared for the patient. The patient's response guides the words to be said and the approach to be taken. What is said in a prepared speech may not concern or interest the patient. It may in fact threaten his self, and he becomes defensive and antagonistic and failure is imminent. The patient should not be criticized or his ideas rejected.

Communication is an interchange of meanings that takes place between people through thoughts, actions, and attitudes. It is how people act, think, feel, and speak. It not only occurs through the use of words but also through the use and movement of the person (body language), which is important as nonverbal communication.

Each person has his own territory, the required size of which is not known. During the first visit the control therapist will designate to the patient the territories that belong to him. These areas will be the sink where the patient cleans his teeth and the area where he will be during the discussion periods. Only once will the control therapist need to indicate to the patient the territory that is his. He will without exception appropriately return to it day after day, week after week, month after month, and year after year. The control therapist will also have her own territories, which will be the positions she takes during the cleaning and discussion periods. The amount of space that each patient requires will vary, and the patient will tell the control therapist in body motion how much room is needed. If the patient stands back, is withdrawn, and is restless, he needs more territory. The control therapist must allow more space. This may mean moving supplies and equipment, but it must be done or the patient will not be comfortable and will be unable to give his full attention to the program. This can happen in reverse, also. The patient may not allow the control therapist sufficient territory, and she becomes uncomfortable and is unable to concentrate on the material to be presented. Again adjustments must be made. As the program progresses and the patient and the control therapist become better acquainted, the distance between the two becomes shorter and shorter until by visits 5 and 6 a close relationship exists that is vital for effective nutritional counseling.

The control therapist must be a good listener. The patient should be allowed to express his desires, his ideas, and his misgivings. He should have the opportunity to participate in decision making. The sessions are discussion periods, not lectures, and the language used is in simple terms and short words. Technical terms should be followed immediately with explanations. All patients should be treated with the same respect regardless of their profession or vocation, their economic and social status, their color or creed. The program should be altered to meet the patient's needs, not his apparent status in life.

There will be times when the control therapist will exchange personal information with the patient. This is important because the patient will not give all without receiving a little. The conversation should be kept at a professional level. Controversial topics such as politics and religion should be avoided.

The Child 2 Years to Preadolescent

A child should never be underestimated. He has tremendous ability to learn and a great desire to please. He is capable at a reasonable age and with his mother's help of preventing dental disease. He will and does teach the parents, if they are willing, how to clean their teeth, as well as his relatives, his friends, and anyone else who will listen. The *program* is the same for children as for adults except that it is altered to meet the needs of a specific age.

The supplies are the same as for the adult, except that he receives a junior size toothbrush, Butler Jr. No. 111 G.U.M. Floss Aids are used by children up to about 7 or 8 years of age.

The visual aids and take-home material are in the form of bright colored pictures. Information to be discussed is presented in visual form. In order to point out large amounts of sugar in the diet, sugar is measured by the spoonful. To learn about eating a well-balanced diet, the child makes a pretend breakfast, lunch, and dinner by arranging plastic food models (Chapter 6) on plates. Filmstrips oriented to the child are also used, for example, *Judy's Family Food Notebook* (Chapter 6). A toy box filled with "Junk," the colorful "take homes," as well as the oral hygiene supplies serve as rewards for children.

It is important to remember that if the child is treated like a child, he will act like a child. If he is treated like an adult, he will act like an adult, and the therapist will have made a friend for life.

The Teen Years

All patients must motivate themselves. The young person from 12 years through late teens must also be considered and treated like an adult. There must be a program, just flossing and brushing will not "turn anyone on," especially the ones in this age group. One should treat him as an intelligent person and respect him for his intelligence. These people are children, but a little older; they too are eager and willing to learn, but learning is more readily accepted if it can become a direct concern to them.

Discussions with the patient give him an opportunity to verbalize and question. Seek information from him, not information that is critical, such as how often he eats sweets, but rather what kind of food the high school cafeteria serves, during what hours, how much does it cost? Can he buy food from machines? Maybe you know the answers, but hear them again. Find out about the ball games, and who is winning them. Ask about his class schedule, if he has good teachers, show him that you care. Use the information he gives you and let him know that you are going to use it. Offer him future help in nutrition classes if this is his need. Be his friend. Do not be critical. State the scientific facts involved in the program; be honest. "Tell it as it is, Charlie Brown."

Do not threaten; he may not care if he gets pimples from eating candy; however, he may wish to have more endurance for track or football. A living example means more to him than what will happen if he doesn't do such and such. Let him observe the shining teeth and the healthy gums of the control therapist. He will be more inclined to want his teeth to be shining too, and he will want it to occur before his senior class pictures are taken, which might be next week. Do not be amazed when this person returns to purchase thirty-six spools of dental floss so he will have plenty when he goes to college.

Perhaps all teenagers will not so respond, but then do all adults? If the control therapist is having 95 to 100 per cent success with adults, she will have the same with teenagers.

The Older Patient

Persons in the upper age levels may state that they are too old to begin such a program, that it is for younger persons. This person is actually asking if he is important enough to be taught. Into the program, these same people will ask, "Why didn't you teach me this long ago?" Another may say, "I don't know if I want to go through all this bother," and in the next instance will criticize previous dentists for taking a look and fixing the teeth without stopping the disease. (In this instance the husband and wife each had six teeth. The husband had gone through the program and had referred his wife for control.)

Nutritional counseling is important for this age group. Their income is less, their food selections are made among the cheaper, soft, refined carbohydrate foods. They are eating less meat, milk, eggs, and fresh fruits and vegetables. Incomes may be adequate for the purchase of foods, but these people are saving for what might lie ahead. Food is the one item they can save on.

In teaching oral hygiene techniques to the elderly and to the handicapped, aids such as the Perio-Aid, Floss Aids, or electric toothbrush (Water Pik) may be necessary. The tools needed will depend upon the physical abilities of the patient.

The Deaf

The control program for the deaf is the same as for the person who is not. The only difference is in the method of communication.

To effectively teach this person, the control therapist must be able to converse with the patient. If she is not trained in sign language or finger spelling, teaching can be accomplished only through writing. The information is written in the presence of the patient as if conversing with a person who can hear. This patient will want to take these written notes home with him so he can reread and study them. Visuals aids are extremely important because a picture or a model can tell many stories. The printed take-home material is of value to deaf people because this is what they rely upon to gain the full understanding of dental disease, its causes and prevention.

Deaf children are like all children. If the material is interesting they will give their attention. If it is presented at their grade level, they will learn. Again, visual aids are necessary in teaching the deaf child. These children respond to warmth and attention and can be a source of great satisfaction.

The Blind

The program is altered to meet the needs of blind patients. Use of tactile aids, such as models with emphasis on the demonstration in the patient's own mouth, in conjunction with verbal discussion is the most effective method of teaching. The blind person is very receptive. His concentration is acute because there are fewer distractions. He wants to be and should be treated like all other persons. Remember, this person is used to his handicap, it is the control therapist who is not.

More time may be required with the program to care for handicapped persons. These people should not be hurried, and shortcuts should not be taken because the future care they give their mouths and even the food they eat may be dependent on what and how they perform during this program.

Occasionally the control therapist should recall the difficult cases with their successful outcomes, remembering how appreciative the people are after having been helped to find ways to help themselves. It is truly a health service that is performed, and it generates a great deal of personal satisfaction. The control therapist has not only gained the respect of a grateful patient but also the respect of the entire dental team and the dental profession as a whole. She has made a direct contribution to the success of the dentist for whom she works and is instrumental in the growth of the dental practice. Perhaps the most gratifying of all are the friends she has made.

3

*The dental staff makes it possible
to accomplish the many tasks and details
that constitute a complete and totally
comprehensive preventive dental practice.*

The Role of the Dental Health Team

The amount of detail given to various functions is dependent upon the available staff. If a more complex approach to a dental practice is attempted by including dental education for the patient, then further organization of the methods and procedures is necessary.

Everyone concerned with the dental program should have a broad interest and capacity to integrate what he is doing with the single purpose of furthering the total concept of serving the dental patient in helping him to control his dental disease.

In every phase of dentistry an alert positive attitude generates more enthusiasm and provides more of a challenge in keeping the profession vital and dynamic.

THE ROLE OF THE RECEPTIONIST

The person who serves as the receptionist must have communicative skills. It is important that she be able to think, speak, and write so that her response informs the patient that he has been heard and understood. Dentistry has much to say to the patient, and it is the receptionist who is the first to open this line of communication.

In her performance of duties, she continually comes into contact with the patient, but she lacks an appreciation of his dental needs as understood by the dentist and the dental assistant. This separation in communication must be overcome so that the entire dental staff views dentistry in the same manner. Personalities and effort must join together to form a strong dental health team.

Of necessity, there is a delegation of duties, but the dentist and the receptionist should strive to work together and discuss patient management. Philosophy and concepts of dentistry should be dealt with to know what can be contributed. All members of the staff must talk to, inform, discuss with, and cooperate with the receptionist to provide her with knowledge of what is actually occurring with the dental patients. It is not a dependency upon others that is being suggested but a free flow of information so that the receptionist is brought into the dental practice.

The receptionist needs to know not only the when of the next appointment but also the why of the control or prevention. A control program will fail if she does not believe in it, and she can only believe in it if she has experienced the change that takes place in her own mouth. With this experience, she can communicate to the patient. She can recommend it to others who seek it.

The efforts of the receptionist are directed to letting the patient know that he has selected the right place to solve the problem that confronts him. The ways in which the patient can be helped are expanded through dental education, but before it can begin it is necessary to set the stage that will make

FIG. 3-1. Receptionist's desk area with Valcom signal system.

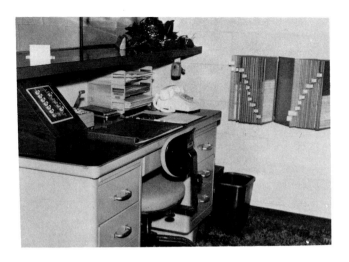

it possible for new concepts to be understood, accepted, and applied.

The continuity of the dental office is maintained by the receptionist as she coordinates and guides the functioning of the dental practice. It is the creativeness of the individual that changes routine procedures into a personalized approach.

Signal System

For effective patient flow with minimal effort in communication, the Valcom light system[1] (Fig. 3-1) is used between staff members to indicate the status of patients. This system is made up of a panel of two rows of signal push buttons that light up in all rooms when the buttons are pressed. Ten seconds after a button is activated an intermittent warning tone will sound until the lights are extinguished by pressing the reset button on any Valcom unit. The white signals on the left of the unit are designated one for each member of the staff. The colored signals on the right are predetermined messages. For example, for the left column, the white signals, from the top down, are designated as the dentist, receptionist, dental assistant, control therapist, and hygienist. The colored signals in the

right column, from the top down, when activated indicate such messages as the patient has arrived, dentist ready, have patient wait, incoming telephone calls, and emergency situations.

The black push button on the bottom right of the control panel produces an audible signal without delay and is used in emergency conditions or when instant communication is desired.

Telephone Procedure

The Receptionist Check List is designed to help guide the receptionist in the care of the patient during the initial period of treatment (Fig. 3-2).

The telephone conversation should be warm and friendly and not hurried. The information offered by the receptionist should reflect the preventive philosophy. Information is obtained at this time so that when the patient arrives at the dental office much of the preliminary information has been acquired and more effort can be made in making the patient feel at home. The first part of the check list is completed with this conversation and an appointment is scheduled.

If this is an appointment for a child and it is his first visit to the dentist, the pamphlet *Child's First Visit* (ADA) is mailed to the parent.

---

[1] Valtronic Corp., 120 E. 144th St., Bronx, N.Y. 10451.

Patient Flow

The flow of patients for diagnostic and control procedures is diagramed by using circles to designate the different rooms in the office. An overall view of patient management will be gained by tracing the patient's movements as indicated by the lines and arrows and reviewing the summary of the procedures that are accomplished by the receptionist at each appointment session.

The procedure for new patients follows. Adult Examination—Phase I (Fig. 3-3; Chap. 7).

A. Appointment time is 30 minutes.

RECEPTIONIST CHECK LIST

Patient _____ Age _____

Address _____
                                                   Zip Code
Telephone _____ Business phone _____

Emergency (chief concern) _____

_____

Appointment scheduled _____

Emergency PBP Acquaintance Form 49A _____

Attitude _____

Insurance Company _____

Welfare, Eligibility Form _____ Signature _____

EXAMINATION   Phase I   Welcome _____

Child Health History PBP Form 91 _____

Cardex Filing System complete _____

Phase II Referral Letter mailed _____: Physician's Letter mailed _____

Phase III Date Diagnosis needed _____: Treatment Plan _____

Fee Estimate _____: Written Diagnosis _____

Disease Control Program   yes _____   no _____

Newsletter mailing list _____

Prophylaxis _____: Fluoride Polish _____: Fluoride _____

Patient treatment planning _____

Financial arrangements _____

Treatment scheduled _____

Recall File _____: Family Recall File _____

FIG. 3-2. Receptionist Check List.

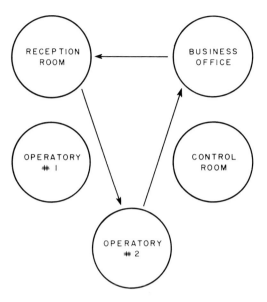

FIG. 3-3. Patient flow — Diagram of Phase I of the examination.

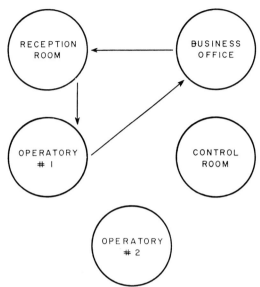

FIG. 3-5. Patient flow — Diagram of Phase II of the examination and Phase III, the consultation appointment.

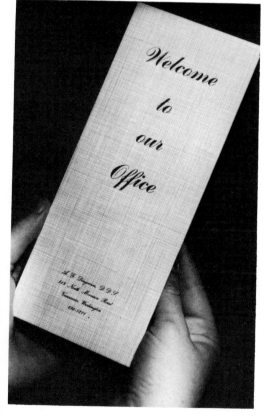

FIG. 3-4. The welcome brochure (adapted from Dr. Robert Barkley).

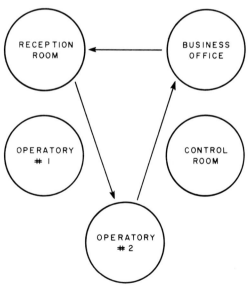

FIG. 3-6. Patient flow — Diagram of the recall examination appointment.

B. The information on the Receptionist Check List is completed through "Appointment scheduled."
C. The health history is part of the examination form — Phase I — and is taken by the receptionist at this time.
D. The *Welcome to Our Office* brochure (Fig. 3-4) is given to the patient. He is asked to read it in the reception room while he waits for the dentist (approximately 10 minutes). The welcome states the philosophy of the dentist and tells the patient that this office cares about him.
E. The patient is taken to operatory no. 2 by the dental assistant.
F. After this phase of the examination, an appointment is made for 2 to 4 days following.

Child's Examination — Phase I:
A. Appointment time is 30 minutes.
B. Child arrives and is greeted by the receptionist.
C. The health history and dental history are completed by the receptionist and the parent (PBP form 91).
D. The patient is taken to operatory no. 2 by the dental assistant.
E. Examination procedures are carried out.
F. The parent or parents are rescheduled for diagnosis. The child is included if he or the dentist desires.

Patient Requiring Emergency Care:
This person should be considered a prospective new patient who will continue on into an examination and treatment after the emergency care. The Professional Budget Plan form 49A is completed.
The health history is listed on the reverse side of this form. The required treatment is performed, and the post-treatment message given.

Adult Examination — Phase II (Fig. 3-5):
A. Appointment time is 30 minutes.
B. The patient is seated in operatory no. 1 by the dental assistant.
C. After the examination, the patient is dismissed to the business office where he reads and signs a health history request letter to his physician.

D. The patient is rescheduled for the consultation appointment.

Adult Examination — Phase III, Consultation Appointment (Fig. 3-5):
A. Appointment time is 30 minutes (15 minutes with the dentist).
B. The patient reads the written diagnosis in the reception room. (It is important to ascertain that the patient can read.)
C. The dentist and the patient discuss the diagnosis in operatory no. 1. Questions are answered.
D. The patient is rescheduled for the disease control program.

Child's Examination — Consultation Appointment:
A. The dentist and parent view the x-ray films and discuss the diagnosis.
B. The child is scheduled for disease control.

The procedure for recall examinations follows (Fig. 3-6; Chapter 9).

Adult Recall Examination:
A. The patient is scheduled for recall examination.
B. If it has been some time since his previous visit, the health history is brought up to date and the *Welcome to Our Office* is given to him to read.

Child's Recall Examination:
A. The patient is scheduled for the recall examination.
B. Recall procedures are conducted, and if the patient is under control, the prophylaxis and fluoride treatments are completed.
C. If the patient displays disease, then Phase II of the children's examination is scheduled for consultation with the parent.

The patient flow for disease control visit 1 is shown in Figure 3-7; for disease control visits 2 through 8, in Figure 3-8. The scheduling for the Disease Control Visits follows.

Visit 1: Time allowed: 30 minutes for the dentist and 1 hour for the control therapist.

Visit 2: The following day. Time allowed: 45 minutes.

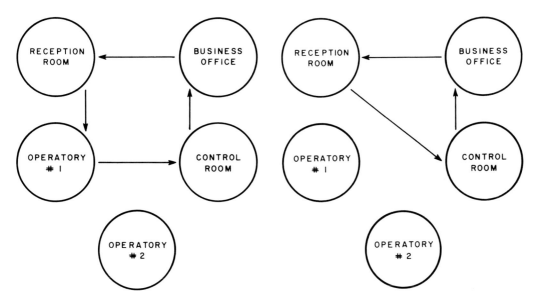

FIG. 3-7. Patient flow—Diagram of disease control visit 1.

FIG. 3-8. Patient flow—Diagram of disease control visits 2 through 8.

Visit 3: The following day or 1 or 2 days later. Time allowed: 1 hour.

Visit 4: The following day. Time allowed: 45 minutes.

Visit 5: The following day or 1 or 2 days later. Time allowed: 1 hour.

Visit 6: Approximately 1 week following visit 5. Time allowed: 1 hour.

Visit 7: Approximately 1 month following visit 6. Time allowed: 30 minutes.

Visit 8: Approximately 2 months following visit 7. Time allowed: 30 minutes.

Scheduling for the Control Program

To avoid confusion, disease control can be color coded. The color of the control program has been designated blue in our office. Appointment cards for the control appointments as well as the recall cards are blue. Appointment cards for dental treatment are white (Fig. 3-11).

Appointments for control are made as convenient as possible for the patient: early morning, lunch hour, after school, or at the end of the work day. A word of caution is necessary: Early morning appointments may seem desirous to the patient but in reality are most difficult to handle. The receptionist should be sensitive to the patient's needs. If the patient is 10 minutes late for an 8:00 A.M. appointment, in all probability it is too early for the patient, and he actually wishes to change to a later time. (Control patients are usually early for their appointments.) A mother may think a before-school appointment is ideal, but it really represents chaos. The scheduling should be flexible.

It is not satisfactory to schedule the patient for both a control visit and a treatment session until after he has completed visit 6 because control visits 1 through 6 are lengthy and involved. If complete patient cooperation is to be obtained, the patient cannot handle treatment during this period.

It should be conveyed to the patient that this is necessary to control the present disease and to insure better restorative treatment. Restorations that are placed in diseased tissue cannot be of the quality that can be achieved when the teeth are clean and the gums are free of infection.

SCHEDULING DISEASE CONTROL PROGRAM
Individual - Age 5 and all years thereafter

30 minutes Doctor	DISEASE CONTROL # 1 Snyder test and vitamin C test Staining Flossing Use of phase microscope Film strip
1 hour Control Therapist	Supplies Dietary instruction Discussion of periodontal disease Brushing technique
45 minutes Following day	DISEASE CONTROL # 2 Flossing and brushing Proper use of Perio-Aid Removal of stains
1 hour Following or 1-2 days later	DISEASE CONTROL # 3 Saliva testing Demonstration of water sprays
45 minutes Following day	DISEASE CONTROL # 4 Discussion of fluoride, decay and x-rays
1 hour Following day	DISEASE CONTROL # 5 Identification and discussion of carbohydrate foods as related to dental disease
1 hour One week later	DISEASE CONTROL # 6 Dietary evaluation and counseling Nutritional counseling with mothers of children 5 years through high school. Time required: 30 minutes

Prophylaxis and fluoride treatment by Doctor or Hygienist. Dental treatment started.

30 minutes One month later	DISEASE CONTROL # 7 Saliva test Supplies
30 minutes Two months later	DISEASE CONTROL # 8 Supplies Recall

FIG. 3-9. Scheduling the disease control program.

SCHEDULING DISEASE CONTROL PROGRAM
Mother and Child ages 2-4 years
(Mother flosses and brushes child's teeth)

30 minutes Doctor	DISEASE CONTROL # 1 - Mother only Snyder test and Vitamin C test Staining Flossing Use of phase microscope Film strip
1 hour Control Therapist	Supplies Dietary instruction Discussion of periodontal disease Brushing technique
1 hour Following day	DISEASE CONTROL # 2 - Mother only Saliva testing Flossing and brushing Proper use of Perio-Aid, Removal of stains
1 hour Following or 1-2 days later	DISEASE CONTROL # 3 - Mother and child Saliva testing for child Demonstration of water sprays
1 hour Following day	DISEASE CONTROL # 4 - Mother and child Discussion of fluoride, decay, x-rays
1 hour 30 minutes Following or 1-2 days later	DISEASE CONTROL # 5 - Mother and child Identification and discussion of carbohydrate foods as related to dental disease
1 hour One week later	DISEASE CONTROL # 6 - Mother only Dietary evaluation and counseling

Prophylaxis, fluoride treatment by Doctor or Hygienist. Dental treatment started

1 hour One month later	DISEASE CONTROL # 7 - Mother and child Saliva tests Supplies
1 hour Two months later	DISEASE CONTROL # 8 - Mother and child Supplies Recall

Fig. 3-10. Scheduling the disease control program for the child with mother.

In scheduling a control visit and a treatment session together, as may be done on visit 7 or 8, the control visit must precede the treatment session. The patient cannot clean his teeth effectively if fluoride has been applied or if his mouth has been anesthetized.

The type of appointment book to be used depends upon the dental practice, and it may require some experimentation to find one that serves the purpose. It seems essential that the control appointments be listed in relationship to the dentist's daily treatment schedule. A book with a three-column day for 6 days shows at a glance the office schedule for the week (Fig. 3-12). From this, the receptionist makes a listing of the next day's appointments on a three-column appointment sheet such as PBP form 112. One column is used for each room—two operatories and one control room. The lists are placed in each room so that each of the staff can preview the day's schedule.

DISEASE CONTROL PROGRAM

NAME_____

VISIT #1_____VISIT #5_____

VISIT #2_____VISIT #6_____

VISIT #3_____VISIT #7_____

VISIT #4_____VISIT #8_____

RECALL VISIT WITH PREVENTIVE NURSE EVERY FOUR MONTHS. RECALL EXAM BY DOCTOR ONCE A YEAR.

ARTHUR GARY DINGERSON, D. D. S.
513 N. MORRISON ROAD   VANCOUVER, WASH. 98664
PHONE 694-5211

IN ORDER TO KEEP YOUR DISEASE UNDER CONTROL, IT IS IMPORTANT THAT YOU RETURN REGULARLY FOR NECESSARY CARE. OUR OFFICE WILL NOTIFY YOU IN ADVANCE AND PLEASE MAKE AN APPOINTMENT AT YOUR EARLIEST POSSIBLE CONVENIENCE. THANK YOU.

JAN._____MAY_____SEPT._____

FEB._____JUNE_____OCT._____

MARCH_____JULY_____NOV._____

APRIL_____AUG._____DEC._____

NAME _____

M _____

ARTHUR GARY DINGERSON. D.D.S.
513 N. MORRISON ROAD   VANCOUVER, WASHINGTON
PHONE 694-5211

MON. _____AT_____   THURS. _____AT_____

TUES. _____AT_____   FRI. _____AT_____

WED. _____AT_____   SAT. _____AT_____

A BROKEN APPOINTMENT IS A LOSS TO EVERYONE. PLEASE INFORM US ONE DAY IN ADVANCE IF YOU ARE UNABLE TO KEEP YOUR APPOINTMENT.

FIG. 3-11. Appointment cards.

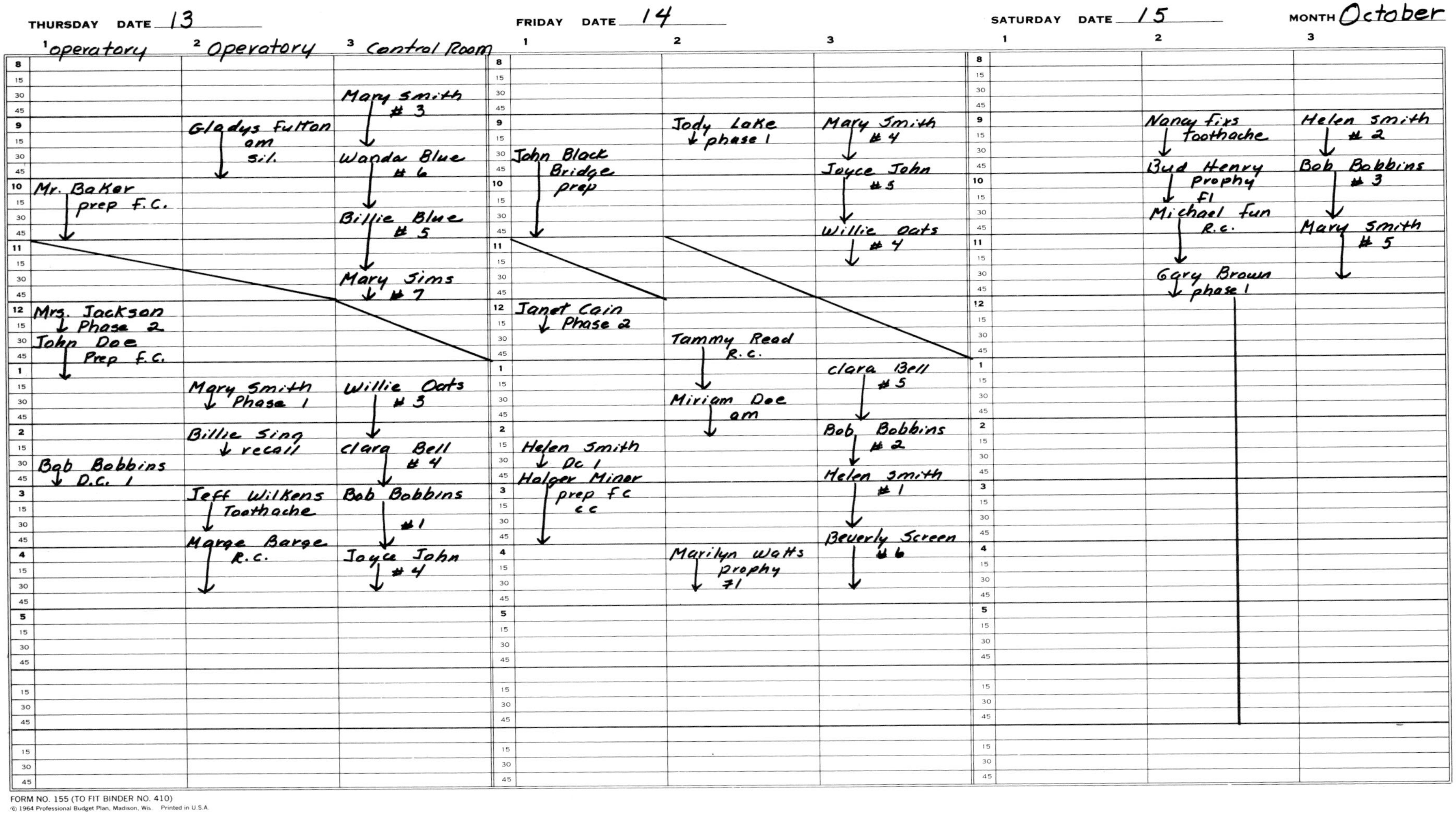

FIG. 3-12. Appointment book PBP form 155.

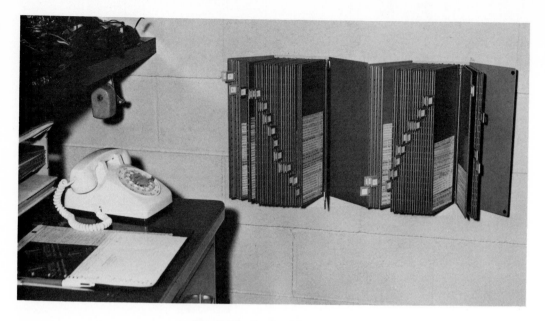

FIG. 3-13. Cardex filing system.

Letter	Phase II	Diag.	Treat Plan	Est.	Phase III	Will Call	Insur. Form	DC	DC #7	Snyder Test	DC #8	Px Fl	Treat	Recall				

Chart #   Name   Telephone   Address

                                                           City   State   Zip

Referred by _____   Health History   Disease Control   Snyder Tests
                                                            1 _____   _____
X-ray _____   _____   2 _____   _____
                                                            3 _____   _____
_____   _____   4 _____   _____
                                                            5 _____   _____
_____   _____   6 _____   _____
                                                            7 _____   _____
Models _____   _____   8 _____   _____

Examination _____   _____

_____   _____

Preference of Payment: Letters   Fluoride Application
Cash in advance, 5% reduction _____   _____   _____
One-third down, balance in six monthly payments _____   _____   _____
One-fourth down, balance in three monthly payments _____   _____   _____
Budget Plan: no down payment with regular monthly
payments and 1% charged on unpaid balance _____   _____   _____
Insurance - name of Company _____   _____   _____
Welfare _____ ID Number _____   _____   _____
Other _____   _____   _____

FIG. 3-14. Front page of patient's chart in a plastic folder, (form adapted from Dr. Robert J. Peshek and PBP).

Patient Record

The patient's complete file is contained within a PBP no. 37 brown envelope. The chart is numbered and placed within the file cabinet. The name, address, and chart number are typed on the identification strip and placed alphabetically according to the patient's last name in the Cardex file (Fig. 3-13). The brown envelope will not leave the filing cabinet again. Rather, the front and back pages of the chart as well as current information are placed in a plastic folder, PBP 162. This becomes the working chart (Fig. 3-14).

The column across the top is used to inform the receptionist of procedures to be carried out. Adhesive stickers are used as signals and are placed under the appropriate item upon the plastic envelope. The front page of the chart provides information concerning the referral of the patient, dates of x-ray examinations, diagnostic models, examinations, and health histories. Pertinent health information such as the presence of diabetes, tuberculosis, and allergies to drugs are recorded in large red letters on the front of the chart.

The dates of the control visits are listed as well as the dates and results of the modified Snyder tests. This indicates to the dental staff the patient's pattern on the control program.

A listing of the dates letters were mailed serves as a reminder of the need for correspondence. A record of fluoride applications informs the dentist at a glance how many times fluoride has been applied. Finally, information listed under the preference of payment is of value to the receptionist in that it informs her of the patient's intent of payment.

The back page of the chart is placed facing outward (Fig. 3-15). It has the treatment plan prepared by the dentist. The work

Name			Chart #		
Units of time	Treatment Plan	Work Schedule for next appointment	Date	Services Rendered	Fee

FIG. 3-15. Back of patient's chart in plastic folder (form adapted from Dr. Robert J. Peshek).

schedule is completed by the chair-side assistant after each treatment. A notation is made on the chart that informs the receptionist the amount of time required for the following appointment. The date, services rendered, and the fee are also filled in by the chair-side assistant or hygienist. The fee is then transposed to the accounting records by the receptionist.

The dental chart is made up of forms used

within a three-appointment examination and is discussed in detail in Chapter 7.

The Physician's Letter (Fig. 3-16) is prepared by the receptionist and signed by the patient at the termination of Phase II (visit 2 of the examination). The recall patient will sign the letter on the second visit.

The purpose of the letter is to determine specific health factors. For example, in patients having had congenital heart defects

Date

Address

Dear Doctor _____,

Regarding Jane E. Doe, a mutual patient, who has been referred to me for dental treatment.

Is her (or his) medical status normal? Is there any pertinent medical history that would have a bearing upon dental treatment?

It is my desire to offer your patient the best dental treatment available.

Thank you for your interest and any inconvenience this request may have put to you.

Sincerely,

A. G. Dingerson, D. D. S.

AGD:md

I have read the above request and ask Dr. _____
to inform Dr. Dingerson of anything he feels would be of benefit in my dental treatment.

Thank you,

Sincerely,

_____

FIG. 3-16. Physician's letter (adapted from Dr. Jerome S. Mittleman).

or degenerative conditions of the heart valves with or without replacement, penicillin or erythromycin would be prescribed 2 days prior to the beginning of the control program and would continue for 2 days after all the bleeding has stopped. This is a treatment time of about 10 days. There may be other conditions present that warrant medical preparation, which can best be determined through correspondence with the physician.

The preventive forms that make up the rest of the chart are used primarily by the control therapist and are discussed in the areas of use in this text.

The Written Diagnosis

The patient's personal diagnosis is given in Phase III or visit 3 of the examination (Chapter 7). It is dictated by the dentist into a tape recorder and then typed for presentation to the patient. It begins with a thought on prevention and its desirability. It continues with a statement of the dentist's philosophy of dentistry and what he personally wants to provide in the way of dental service. It is a written recap of the examination check list. Treatment recommendations as well as treatment limitations are listed. The prognosis of the present conditions as ef-

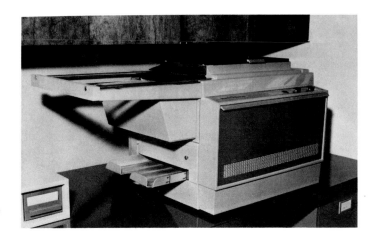

FIG. 3-17. The Apēco copy machine.

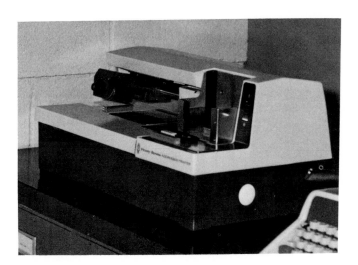

FIG. 3-18. An addresser (Pitney Bowes).

fected by disease control and restorative treatment are discussed.

The basic format of this diagnosis is established and made up in the form of master sheets. The material used is adjusted to each patient and becomes individually tailored as it is dictated on tape.

Master Sheets

These are original sheets from which copies are made. They include informational material, letters, charts, and forms. To have the material composed simplifies procedures and serves as a beginning in the communication with the patient. As changes occur the forms and messages can readily be changed.

To enable the dental practice to be creative and responsive, some means of processing printed material economically is necessary. This can be accomplished through use of a copy machine (Fig. 3-17). An addresser is used to address correspondence (Fig. 3-18), which helps relieve the receptionist from a time-consuming duty so that more of her effort may be directly related to people.

Letters for Prevention

The preventive practice communicates with its patients, and one source of communication is through correspondence. Each letter is personalized and typed individually to meet the personality of the patient.

The dental hygienist or the control therapist indicates which letter from the master sheets is to be used so that appropriate information will be included. These letters are primarily reports of test results, congratulations extended upon completion of visits, and thank-you letters.

The disease control letter to Tammy (Fig. 3-19) is reporting the results of her Snyder test. This letter states the results and what it means in terms of the number of bacteria. It compares the oral environment of now with that of 6 months ago, and it reiterates what to do to keep the test results low and to maintain favorable results.

Date

Address

Dear Tammy,

    Congratulations! Your recent Snyder Test was negative indicating that at this time the number of bacteria that can cause decay in your mouth is negligible. This is an improvement over the Snyder Test taken six months ago which was a 2+.

    The number of bacteria is now determined by the effectiveness of your flossing and brushing technique as well as the amount of refined carbohydrates you are eating in your selection of foods. Keep up these good habits.

    GOOD FLOSSING!
                    GOOD BRUSHING!

                            Sincerely,

                            Marilyn Dingerson
                            Disease Control Therapist

FIG. 3-19. Disease control letter stating the results of a Snyder test.

A Disease Control Program Completion letter (Fig. 3-20) is typed for each patient who completes the control program. It praises him for his participation; it states what the program included and what he must do to benefit further from it. Lastly, it thanks him for his cooperation and states that the office staff looks forward to seeing him again. The completion letter is modified for the child and adapted to the person to whom it will be sent.

The Preventive Newsletter

Another facet in communication with the patient is the monthly newsletter. The newsletter, *The Prevention Key* (Fig. 3-21) is sent only to those who have gone on to the control program. Its purpose is to provide additional information about oral health, control, and prevention and tells the patient we are thinking of him. It is also hoped that it will reinforce what has been presented in the dental office so that it will carry over into the home. *The Key* is reproduced by the copy machine, and the addresser is used to address the envelopes in which it is sent.

Financial Arrangements

The fee for the control program is charged on control visit 1; there is no charge for the remaining visits. It is important that this be explained to the patient. The control program in this text is a specific program with a set number of appointments and a set fee; the program is identical for all patients with only alterations made to fit individual needs. By making the charge on the first visit, the patient cannot save money by not coming in or canceling; he will, in fact, be wasting money, as well as an opportunity, if he does not avail himself of the visits offered in his behalf. The patient spends a minimum of 30 minutes with the dentist, plus 1 hour with the control therapist on the first visit. Time alone justifies the fee. The fee charged for the program is insignificant when compared to the potential of its application.

The financial arrangements for the treatment planned are made with the patient following the prophylaxis and fluoride treatment. This is the appointment following disease control visit 6. These arrangements are made at this time and not before because

---

Address

Dear _____,

    Congratulations on completing the Disease Control Program.

    Effective home care of the mouth can never be over-emphasized. We have gone through the details of flossing, brushing, food intake, food selection, and nutrition.

    It is important that you continue to apply the skills and knowledge that you have received to maintain the health and appearance of the structures of your mouth.

    Thank you for your cooperation and we all are looking forward to serving you in the future.

                Sincerely,

                Dr. A. G. Dingerson

AGD:md

FIG. 3-20. Disease Control Program Completion Letter.

the patient has learned about himself and can *now* make a knowledgeable decision concerning his mouth. Some patients will make arrangements following diagnosis, and this is acceptable.

The treatment plan is used in making appointments for further care.

Post-treatment Information Messages

These printed messages are written by the dentist and produced by the receptionist from master sheets that are processed through the copy machine and cut to proper size (Fig. 3-22). They are given to the patient

as an explanation of dental procedures, follow-up care, and background information of the treatment that was carried out at that specific visit. They are stored in the operatories and are given to the patient by the chair-side assistant. The treatment messages used are:

Oral examination
Cleaning of the teeth
Fluoride
Full survey of x-rays
Caries-detecting x-rays
Diagnostic models
Root canal therapy

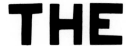 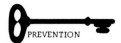

THE ⚷ PREVENTION ⚷ KEY

Vol. 1 No. 1   January 1973

A. G. Dingerson, D. D. S.
513 N. Morrison Road
Vancouver, Washington 98664

The idea of Prevention and its effect on health is of value not only to preserve the mouth, but also a person's well being. Much is being said about environment in our society today. An upgrading of the care of the mouth as you have experienced is definitely contributing to the elimination of unwanted bacteria and their waste products. A person who practices prevention is doing much to control his environment as well as his future health. These newsletters are designed to inform you of research and studies which you can apply to yourself and your family.

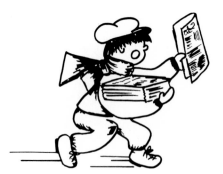

NOTES FROM THE NEWS

CHEWING APPLES AND DENTAL PLAQUE
    No significant cleaning effect attributable to apple-chewing was noted.
        Dent. Pract. and Dent. Rec., 21:194; 1971

DENTAL PLAQUE AND PERIODONTAL DISEASE
    It is recommended that effective methods of plaque control be instituted as a part of the treatment plan for every patient.
        J. Amer. Dent. Hyg. Assoc. 45:186; 1971

FIG. 3-21. *The Prevention Key* newsletter (created by Mrs. Nancy Kennedy, C.D.A.).

Pulpotomy

Amalgam

Plastic or tooth color restorations

Equilibration

Stainless steel crown

Preparation for a gold restoration or gold and porcelain crown or both

Insertion of crown

Preparation of fixed bridge

Insertion of fixed bridge

Extraction

Extraction of impacted wisdom tooth

Insertion of removable partial denture

Preventive examination

Snyder test

Vitamin C test

Ceramco crown

Indirect pulp capping

The Recall System

The recall system consists of a Patient's Recall File set up according to months and a Family Recall File arranged in alphabetical order (Fig. 3-23).

The recall cards are filed at the time of the prophylaxis. The purpose of the Family Recall File is to list all the members of the family in one place and to determine easily when they are due for recall appointments. It is listed as either a recall examination by the dentist or a disease control visit by the control therapist. Very often a patient will want to know when other members of the family are due to be seen. This card provides that information to the receptionist. The family members are identified by number. The patient number and the abbreviated service are placed in the specified month on the Family Recall File.

The System in Operation. At the beginning of the current month the Patient's Recall Card is removed and placed into a call file. After the patient is contacted and an appointment made, the card is placed in the patient's chart. If the patient cannot be reached by phone or mail, the card is dated and replaced in the recall system at the next due date. If the patient does not respond to this notification, the recall card is placed in the dentist's file for review by him.

Changes in appointments are noted on the Family Recall File, and the new appointment is circled in red. If this appointment is not completed, then the Patient's Recall Card is placed in the dentist's file for review.

When the appointment is kept and the services are completed, the next due date is listed on the Patient's Recall Card and it is reentered into the proper monthly file date. The date is marked off the Family Recall File with a line and new dates are posted.

Lastly in the duties of the receptionist, she should be able to assist with the control program during emergencies. She should be able to make the Snyder media, order supplies, and be knowledgeable in the affairs of the office and its overall function.

Dr. A. G. Dingerson
513 N. Morrison Rd.
Vancouver, Washington 98664
Telephone 694-5211

CLEANING OF THE TEETH

To my patients:

Today your teeth were cleaned with the use of ultrasonic and hand instruments and polished with a rubber cup and a fluoride polishing agent.

The tartar that was removed does not produce dental disease. It is, however, a mechanical irritant to the gum tissue and a base for the living bacteria to cling. The dental plaque is the organized bacteria and it is their waste products that produce disease of the teeth and gums.

Twenty-four hours after cleaning the teeth, the dental plaque is reorganized on the hard surfaces in the mouth. So, it is necessary that you clean all surfaces of the teeth, fillings and replacements once a day. There is only one person who can stop dental disease and this is YOU.

FIG. 3-22. An example of a master sheet (adapted from Dr. Robert J. Peshek).

FAMILY RECALL FILE

File Name_____ Phone_____   Family Members   Chart No's.

Address_____ Bus. Phone_____   1._____

_____   2._____

Doctor's recall exam = D.R.E.   3._____

Disease Control + No. = D.C. 7 or 8, etc.   4._____

Preventive Nurse Recall = P.N.R.   5._____

Red circle any Rescheduled dates   6._____

YEAR	JAN.	FEB.	MARCH	APRIL	MAY	JUNE	JULY	AUG.	SEPT.	OCT.	NOV.	DEC.

PIONEER PTG. 1M 7-71

Name_____   Chart No._____

File Name_____ Best Appt. time_____

Address_____ Phone_____ Best time to call_____

_____ Bus. Phone_____ Best time to call_____

Doctor's Review._____

RECALL DATE	UNITS	TREATMENT	REMARKS OR APPOINTMENT DATE

PIONEER PTG. 1M 7-71

FIG. 3-23. Recall file cards (adapted from Dr. Richard Klein and Dr. Ralph O'Connor).

THE ROLE OF THE
DENTAL ASSISTANT

The expansion of the duties adds to the growing capabilities for this position. It is a natural development that these duties now include assistance in carrying out the disease control program as well as in conducting tests that are related to the program. The Certified Dental Assistant gives much support to the program on a routine basis by providing many services.

In the preparation of trays, the instruments are coded with colored tape to designate the various tray setups, such as blue to represent the tray used for disease control visit 1, part A. Pictures showing the instruments on the tray make tray preparation easier and help other members of the staff prepare trays when necessary (Fig. 3-24).

Without the chair-side assistant, the examination procedures that are carried out in Phase II become an impossible task. In every procedure that the dentist accomplishes, it is the chair-side assistant who not only makes dentistry happen but provides that extra touch that gives excellence. Besides assisting the dentist, she serves as a back-up assistant to the control therapist. She may see control patients during emergencies and assist with patient overload during peak hours, such as after school.

Fabrication of Diagnostic Models

Diagnostic models are used in patient diagnosis (Chapter 7) and in the teaching of oral hygiene techniques (Chapters 5 and 8).

In production of a model the correct volume of water for the amount of stone used is placed in a rubber bowl. The bowl containing the water is placed on a diet scale and the calibration set at 0. The correct amount of stone is added by weight. The mix is spatulated, shaken vigorously, and poured into the impression.

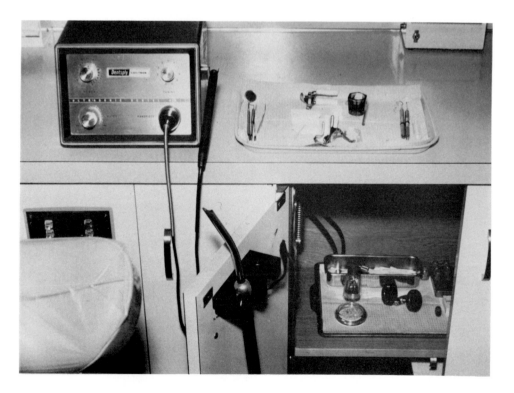

FIG. 3-24. A tray setup in a treatment operatory. The lower shelf extends outward and upward for easy access.

After recovery of the models, any defects are corrected and the models are trimmed on the model trimmer.

Fast-setting impression plaster is placed on the articulator's lower mounting ring, and the lower model is positioned on the plaster so that the occlusal plane is in proper relationship to the articulator. After the lower model has set, the upper model is occluded to the lower model, and the top arm of the articulator with the mounting ring is closed and fastened with impression plaster.

The mounted models are removed from the articulator, and stone is applied over the impression plaster to make a smooth base. After this has hardened, the models are soaked in model gloss, washed off, polished, and remounted on the articulator (Fig. 3-25).

Preparation of Snyder Medium

The Snyder test is discussed in Chapter 4.
Equipment:
Heating element
1-quart sauce pan
Autoclave
Tongue blades
Test tube forceps
Small funnel
Refrigerator
250 ml. distilled water
15 grams Snyder medium
50 unsterile test tubes
4-by-4-inch paper for covering tubes
Rubber bands
Containers (jars) for test tubes
Mesh wire to hold test tubes upright in autoclave tray
Preparation:
Suspend 15 grams of dry material in 250 ml. of distilled water. This is one-fourth the amount suggested on the label. Boil for 1 minute, stirring frequently with the tongue blade to prevent scorching. Dispense approximately 1¼ inches of medium into unsterile test tubes. Place wire mesh in autoclave tray. Place the test tubes within the wire mesh. Place on the side of the tray the pieces of paper that will be used to cover the

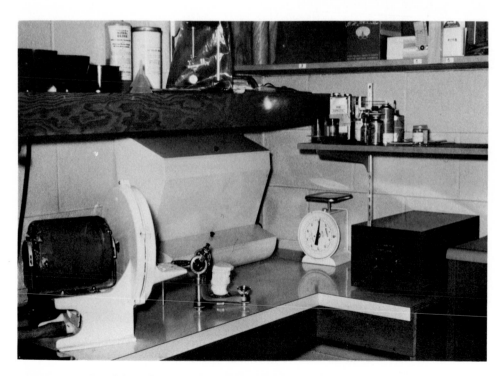

FIG. 3-25. The mounting of diagnostic models on the articulator.

ITEM		BRAND NAME		SUPPLIER		CODE No.	

UNIT (BOX, CASE, CARTON, PACKAGE, BOTTLE, CAN)		QUANTITY TO ORDER FOR BEST PRICE		WHEN TO ORDER — HOW MANY UNITS REMAIN	

DATE	RECEIVED	ISSUED	BALANCE	COST

PIONEER PTG 500 9-70

FIG. 3-26. Inventory supply card (adapted from Dr. Robert J. Peshek).

test tubes after they have been autoclaved. Autoclave at 118° to 121° C. (12 to 15 pounds of steam pressure) for 15 minutes. Remove, allow to cool. Wrap the open end of the test tube with the 4-by-4-inch papers, fasten with rubber bands, and refrigerate.

The Supply System

The purpose of a supply system is to know the supplies that are on hand and to know at which point to reorder so that supplies will always be available. The equipment needed is an inventory card file, colored tags to denote the order point of an item, and signals to indicate the status of the item when it is being procured.

The inventory supply card lists the item, the brand name, the supplier, and the section of storage where it can be found as well as other pertinent information (Fig. 3-26). The name of the item on this card should be the correct name so that in reordering the inventory supply card can be readily identified. If the location of the item is indicated on the card, an article can be located rapidly and with ease. The inventory supply cards are filed in alphabetical order within a filing system.

The reorder tags can be made of heavy paper in any color. They are fastened by means of tape or rubber bands to articles at the point of reorder.

Signals are used on the inventory supply cards to indicate the status of the order. A red signal indicates the item is to be returned, blue indicates it has been ordered, and green shows that it has been back-ordered by the supply company.

It is convenient to have a cabinet or file to hold invoices, packing slips, information concerning orders, catalogs, and other general information in the supply area.

In the placement of supplies, the storage area should be sectioned according to the general use of the merchandise, for example, Section 1—Operative; Section 2—Preventive; Section 3—Laboratory; Section 4—Clerical; Section 5—Office Maintenance; Section 6—Miscellaneous. Figure 3-27 shows a supply area.

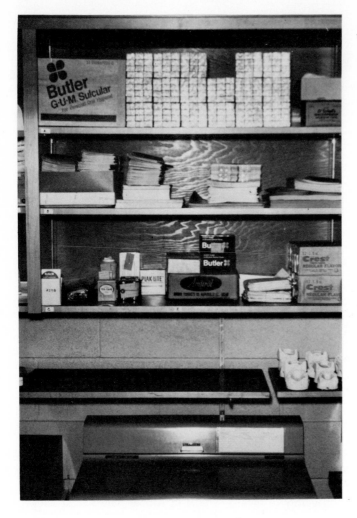

FIG. 3-27. Supply area preventive section.

Purchasing supplies can be enjoyable. It must be done in an orderly fashion; to overstock can be as wasteful as to understock. Each office determines the amounts and the place of purchase. A useful service is the Digest of Discount Dental Supplies,[1] a listing published quarterly. It provides product description at the best price. The information is derived from forty catalogs of dental suppliers.

Ordering Supplies. The wanted item is placed in a want-list notebook. Once a week the supplies are ordered. The inventory

_____
[1] P.O. Box 2176, Ann Arbor, Mich. 48103.

supply card is marked and the blue signal attached.

Receiving Supplies. The items are unpacked and checked against the invoice. The invoice or credit slip is placed in the section of the cabinet for invoices. The signals are removed from the inventory supply card, and the item is crossed off the want list. The item itself is placed in its proper location on the supply shelf with the reorder tag in a place denoting the point to reorder.

Returning Merchandise. The item to be returned is placed in the designated area, and the red signal is placed on the inventory supply card.

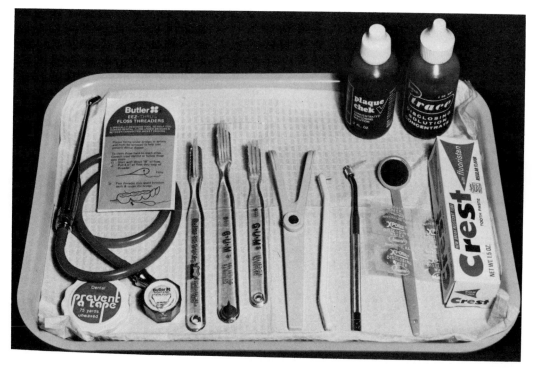

FIG. 3-28. Prevention supplies.

Preventive Inventory

The supplies listed are those used in this text and are but a few of available supplies (Fig. 3-28). Each office will have its preference, which will be determined through results, availability, and cost.

1. Supplies for Testing:
   Disposable Culture Tubes
   Local scientific or medical supply houses or
   Fisher Scientific,
   Fair Lawn, N.J.
   Snyder Media
   Local scientific supply houses or
   Difco Laboratories
   920 Henry St.
   Detroit, Mich.
   Lingual Ascorbic Acid Test — Pro-C Kit
   50 C Brook Ave.
   Deer Park, L.I., N.Y. 11729
   To prepare the solution in the office, dissolve 120 mg. (weighed with an analytical balance) of N/340 2,6-dichlor-oindophenol sodium salt[1] or sodium 2,6 dichlorobenzenoneoindophenol[2] in 50 cc. of absolute methyl alcohol. Using a pipette, place 1 cc. of solution in 50 containers (10 cc. glass or plastic) and air dry. After the methyl alcohol has evaporated, cap container and place in a dry dark place. For use, add 5 cc. distilled water and shake until dissolved. Store in dark and discard after 1 week.
   D-K Caries Activity Test
   D-K Corp.
   3430 East Highland Ave.
   Phoenix, Ariz. 85018
   Fifteen-Minute Caries Conduciveness Test
   G. W. Rapp, Ph.D.
   Professor and Chairman
   Dept. of Biochemistry

---

[1] Available from Eastman Organic Chemicals, Distillation Products Industries, Rochester, N.Y.
[2] Available from Fisher Scientific Co., Fair Lawn, N.J.

Loyola University School of Dentistry
2160 South First Ave.
Maywood, Ill. 60153
Acid and Alkaline Phosphatase Tests
Warner-Chilcott Laboratories
201 Tabor Rd.
Morris Plains, N.J. 07950
Tes-Tape
Local pharmacies or
Eli Lilly and Co.
P.O. Box 618
Indianapolis, Ind. 46206
Young's Caries Etiology Kit
Young Dental Manufacturing Co.
2418 Northline Industrial Blvd.
Maryland Heights, Mo. 63043

2. Nutrition:
Dietronics: Medical Data Processing
P.O. Box 35
Northridge, Calif. 91324

3. Toothbrushes:
Butler Jr. G.U.M. 111
Adult G.U.M. 411
Sulcus G.U.M. 210
Proxabrush handle with brush cores No.
614, 618, and 620
John O. Butler Co.
540 N. Lake Shore Drive
Chicago, Ill. 60611
POH toothbrushes
POH.
P.O. Box 45623
6847 E. 40th St.
Tulsa, Okla. 74145
Electric toothbrush
Water Pik
Teledyne Aqua Tec
1730 East Prospect St.
Fort Collins, Colo. 80521

4. Dental Floss:
Butler unwaxed 50 yards per spool
John O. Butler Co.
540 N. Lake Shore Drive
Chicago, Ill. 60611
Prevent a Tape
P.O. Box 87
Portland, Oreg. 97201

5. Floss Holders:
Floss Aid

Floss Aid Co.
P.O. Box 624
369 Mathew Ave.
Santa Clara, Calif. 95052
Floss-Span
Texell Products Co.
3 Asbury Place
Houston, Tex. 77007

6. Perio-Aids: #1, #2, #3
Marquis Dental Manufacturing Co.
2005 E. 17th Ave.
Denver, Colo. 80206
Toothpicks for use in the Perio-Aid or
Proxabrush handle
World's Fair Toothpick
Available in local supermarkets or
Semantodontics, Inc.
P.O. Box 15668
Phoenix, Ariz. 85018

7. Floss Threaders:
EEZ-Thru Floss Threader
John O. Butler Co.
540 N. Lake Shore Drive
Chicago, Ill. 60611
E Z Flex Floss Threader
Tri Arc Productions
P.O. Box 8055
Tampa, Fla. 33604
Ex-Plac
Preventive Dentistry Products
P.O. Box 754
Corona del Mar, Calif. 92625
Floss Caddy
POH
P.O. Box 45623
6847 E. 40th St.
Tulsa, Okla. 74145

8. Disclosants:
Xpose Disclosing Wafers
Amurol Products Co.
1200 E. Chicago Ave.
Naperville, Ill. 60540
POH Disclosing Wafers
POH
P.O. Box 45623
6847 E. 40th St.
Tulsa, Okla. 74145
Dis-plaque—A two-color dye, liquid or
tablet

Pacemaker Corp.
P.O. Box 16163
Portland, Oreg. 97216
Trace Disclosing Solution
The Lorvic Corp.
8810 Frost Ave.
St. Louis, Mo. 63134
Laclede Disclosing Swabs
Peter, Strong & Co.
415 Lexington Ave.
New York, N.Y. 10017
Plaque Chek Disclosing Solution
Hu-Friedy Mfg. Co.
3118 N. Rockwell St.
Chicago, Ill. 60618
Plak-Lite
International Pharmaceutical Corp.
400 Valley Road
Warrington, Pa. 18976

9. Toothpaste:
Crest professional size
Procter & Gamble Co.
Professional Services Division
Winton Hill Technical Center
Cincinnati, Ohio 45224

10. Mirrors:
Patient mouth mirrors
Procter & Gamble Co.
Professional Services Division
Winton Hill Technical Center
Cincinnati, Ohio 45224
Oral-Lite
PBP
P.O. Box 949
West Beltline Hwy.
Madison, Wis. 53701
Conduct-A-Lite
Semantodontics
P.O. Box 15668
Phoenix, Ariz. 85018
Magnifying mirrors
Floxite Co.
Niagara Falls, N.Y. 14303

11. Makeup Mirrors:
Available through local department,
variety, or drug stores or
JAFCO
17500 South Center Parkway
Andover Industrial Park
Tukwila, Wash. 98124

12. Water Sprays:
Faucet attachment, continuous water flow
POH
P.O. Box 45623
6847 E. 40th St.
Tulsa, Okla. 74145
Dento-Spray
Texell Products Co.
3 Asbury Place
Houston, Tex. 77007
Faucet attachment intermittent water flow
Pulsar
Norcliff Laboratories
Fairfield, Conn. 06430
Unit, intermittent water flow
Water Pik
Teledyne Aqua Tec
1730 East Prospect St.
Fort Collins, Colo. 80521

13. Teeth Models (Write for catalogs):
Columbia Dentoform Corp.
49 East 21st St.
New York, N.Y. 10010
or
PBP
P.O. Box 949
West Beltline Hwy.
Madison, Wis. 53701

14. Food Models: (Write for catalog)
NASCO
Fort Atkinson, Wis. 53538
or
Modesto, Calif. 95352

15. Miscellaneous Items, Oral Hygiene:
Glass slides
Coverslips
Timer for testing
Flashlights—two
Batteries and bulbs
Towels for hand drying
Facial tissue
Cotton applicators
Distilled water in a dropper bottle
Stopwatch
Patient hand mirror
Patient drinking cups
Patient's chest towels and neck clips
Soap dispenser

Vaseline or Borofax for lips
Ajax and mirror cleaners
16. Wall Posters:
Shield of Good Health
    Wheat Flour Institute
    14 East Jackson Blvd.
    Chicago, Ill. 60604
        Write for catalog
Your Snacks: Chance or Choice?
and
A Guide to Good Eating
    National Dairy Council
    111 N. Canal St.
    Chicago, Ill. 60606
Vitamins and Your Body
    Vitamin Information Bureau
    575 Lexington Ave.
    New York, N.Y. 10022
        Write for price list
17. Filmstrips:
Secrets of the Little World
Professional Education and Research,
4130 Farnam St.
Omaha, Nebr. 68131
or
How to Stop Dental Disease
A. V. Scientific Aids, Inc.
639 North Fairfax Ave.
Los Angeles, Calif. 90036
Judy's Family Food Notebook
    Wheat Flour Institute
    14 East Jackson Blvd.
    Chicago, Ill. 60604
Vitamins and You
    Vitamin Information Bureau
    575 Lexington Ave.
    New York, N.Y. 10022
18. Pictures Used in Discussions:
Tablet Test
    Procter & Gamble Co.
    Professional Services Division
    Winton Hill Technical Center
    Cincinnati, Ohio 45224
19. Other Visual Aids:
Plackey Cube
    Plackey Learning Systems
    P.O. Box DE
    Pacific Grove, Calif. 93950

Illustrations in Chapter 4
    Progression of periodontal disease
    (Fig. 4-4)
    Progression of dental decay (Fig. 4-1)
Illustrations in Chapter 5
Patient's x-rays and diagnostic models
20. Informational Material on Oral Hygiene
to Be Taken Home:
Research Explores Plaque
    Superintendent of Documents
    Attn: Customer Service Section
    Government Printing Office
    Washington, D.C. 20402
Personal Oral Hygiene Instruction Sheet
(Write for order form)
POH.
    P.O. Box 45623
    6847 E. 40th St.
    Tulsa, Okla. 74145
A New Plan to Keep Your Teeth for a
Lifetime
and
Is Your Family Missing Out on Fluoride
Protection? (Write for order form)
    Procter & Gamble Co.
    Professional Services Division
    Winton Hill Technical Center
    Cincinnati, Ohio 45224
What You Need to Know and Do to
Prevent Dental Caries (Tooth Decay)
and Periodontal Disease (Pyorrhea)
    Dr. E. A. Pearson, Jr.
    Director, Dental Health Division
    North Carolina State Board of Health
    P.O. Box 2091
    Raleigh, N.C. 27602
21. List of Supplies that the patient will
need and the procedure you wish the
patient to follow during the first several
weeks on this program
22. Prescription Pads for fluoride supplementation
23. Informational Material on Nutrition to
Be Taken Home.
A Guide to Good Eating
Your Snacks: Chance or Choice?
Your Food: Chance or Choice?
A Boy and His Physique

A Girl and Her Figure
National Dairy Council
111 N. Canal St.
Chicago, Ill. 60606

How Do You Score on Nutrition?
Vitamin Information Bureau,
575 Lexington Ave.
New York, N.Y. 10022

Hidden Sugar: Carbohydrate Evaluation Chapter 6.

What Should I Eat? (Foods to Eat Liberally) Chapter 6

What Should I Eat? (Foods to Avoid— Cariogenic—Decay Producing Foods) Chapter 6

24. Work Sheets (in Chapter 6):
Five-day Food Diary
Preventive Measures for Your Dental Health
Diet Evaluation

25. Secretarial Supplies:
Appointment book for control room
Appointment cards
School Excuses
Colored pens, red, blue or black
Pencils, erasers
Patient charts and records

THE ROLE OF THE DENTAL HYGIENIST

We have not had personal experience in working with a dental hygienist as a member of the dental health team. A reflection of what might be considered important to the hygienist is offered in the light of this limitation.

The dental hygienist is expanding her role by acquiring more technical skills in the treatment of dental disease. This increases the potential for serving more people by clinical methods. Every effort should be made to further develop an understanding of the concepts of prevention and the ability to apply measures of control to dental disease. Limiting the field of dental hygiene to clinical procedures is a narrow approach to a complex and interesting challenge.

Dental education of the patient has been a primary function of the dental hygienist. Too elementary an approach achieves elementary results. Applying basic dental sciences is more rewarding than not being knowledgeable of the realities in which we are concerned. Dentistry has much to offer, and the dental hygienist is well equipped to implement new and imaginative approaches to combating dental disease.

A learning process with preventive dentistry concepts, discovering the needs of people, and being able to relate to each patient comes through experience, and this experience must be sought. To reach this goal the dental hygienist cannot delegate dental education to other assistants but must learn by doing. After this stage, a supervisory capacity would be possible, but if the procedures are not continually carried out with patients, growth in this field, as in any other field, stops. Each day new things are learned. When it is felt that everything one needs to know about preventive dentistry is mastered, no further advancement is possible, and failure is at hand.

Is not the control program the role of the dental hygienist?

PART II
The Concepts

*In order to conquer an enemy,
it is wise to first consider its
weaknesses and then its strength.
By communicating a workable
strategy, the attack upon
dental disease will be enhanced.*

Understanding the Mechanism of Dental Disease

THE DISEASE PROCESS

Bacteria colonize around the tooth, below the gum surface, and in the grooves of the teeth. Sucrose (sugar) has been implicated as one of the main sources of energy for the bacteria that reside or cling directly onto the enamel surface. It is the bacterial waste products in the form of acids, which are considered to be the causative agent, that dissolve the tooth structure to form in time a carious lesion. The acid that is formed as the end product of the metabolic cycle of the bacteria etches away on the surface of the tooth, thus beginning the process of decay. As the process continues hour after hour, day after day, and week after week, further destruction can eventually invade the living viable part of the tooth to cause the death of the tooth and the formation of an abscess (Fig. 4-1).

There appears to be a relationship between the well-organized accumulation of bacteria on the tooth and decay. This formation is known as plaque, microbiota, or microcosm, meaning "little world." The inhabitants in the dental plaque are eating, living, and reproducing in an environment that is conducive to their presence but destructive to the host.

In the mouth there are many different types of bacteria. It has often been referred to as the oral museum of bacteriology. The warm moist conditions within the mouth promote their growth. Present over the surface of the mouth is a layer of material in the form of slime that can be felt with the tongue. This has been termed the zoogloea. This coating extends over the mucous membranes, onto the gingival crest, into the gingival sulcus, and over tooth structure, fillings, partials, bridges, and dentures. It is within this gelatinous media that bacteria thrive.

The bacterial population changes or matures if left undisturbed, one type of bacteria suppressing or superseding another. Other bacteria produce materials to be used

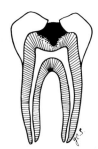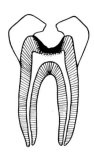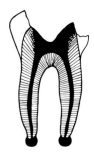

FIG. 4-1. Progression of dental decay (adapted from the American Dental Association).

to support growth of still other bacteria. The longer they are allowed to remain undisturbed, the more organized and more firmly attached they become. These highly organized gummy bacterial masses are held together and isolated from the saliva by a covering called dextran. This is an extracellular polysaccharide that is produced by the action of bacteria on sucrose; long glucose chains are formed. This material serves as a protection from outside influences, it furnishes a food supply for this little world, and it helps hold the plaque together.

The coronal bacteria are sustained in part from the sugar that is consumed and benefit from both quantity and frequency of intake. Refined sugars pass readily through the semipermeable membrane of dextran, but saliva is excluded. The role that saliva plays is under study. It appears that an adequate amount of saliva is necessary and does help to neutralize the acids produced by the bacteria. The saliva is also considered to be bacteriostatic and limits or inhibits the effectiveness of the bacteria. The bacteria just do not do well in the saliva itself, and they need the protection of the gummy bacterial plaque. A deficiency of saliva in amount and quality appears to increase the susceptibility of teeth to decay.

Plaque formation is accentuated in areas of stagnation such as around dental restorations, between teeth, on crowded teeth that are not in harmony with their surroundings, and in mouths that have been neglected or parts that have been missed in oral hygiene procedures. The amount of plaque and its distribution vary greatly in different individuals because of variations in local conditions.

Whether a cavity produced is a smooth surface, pit and fissure, on a root surface, or within the dentin, to the patient it is a defect or, as he often refers to it, a "hole" in his tooth. With the great number and type of bacteria in the mouth, it is difficult for the dentist to determine whether the gluelike material all over the teeth consists of Strep-

tococci, Lactobacilli, or Actinomyces. The important consideration is that what is observed is in fact bacteria and that they are a part of an infectious disease—dental decay.

Periodontal disease, another form caused by bacteria, is produced by toxins emitted from the bacteria in the gingival sulcus or underneath the gum tissue. These toxins appear to have a high plaque pH, or are basic in nature, in contrast to the low pH, or acid, associated with decay.

The bacteria live fairly sheltered lives underneath the gum tissue that surrounds the tooth. They homestead and become more mature and complex as the conditions change that promote bacterial development. The toxins produce tissue breakdown or denuding of the outer layer of tissue covering the gingivae, or gums. This is observed in the mouth and can be detected by noting the red condition of the gums and the areas of bleeding within the sulcus when it is touched with a periodontal probe. The absence of this protective layer of gingiva allows serum to flow freely out into the crevice where the bacteria can utilize this for their food supply. The exudate also includes epithelial cells and is an attractive fare for bacteria. The more successful the bacteria are, the more toxins they produce, which in turn increase the release of more nutrients. As the process continues, the tissues become more inflamed, and puffy, which in effect makes more room for the increasing number of bacteria.

Finally the membranes of the internal portion of the gingival sulcus become so devoid of protection that a state is achieved that allows the bacteria to exist and thrive in an environment similar to that of living inside of the host's body rather than in the oral cavity. At this point the bacteria can readily receive their nourishment directly from the open wounds around the teeth. As long as these conditions persist, the bacteria can continually receive their nutrients from the gums.

The illustration of the mechanism of dental disease depicts the presence of bac-

FIG. 4-2. The mechanism of disease (adapted from the works of Dr. Sumter Arnim).

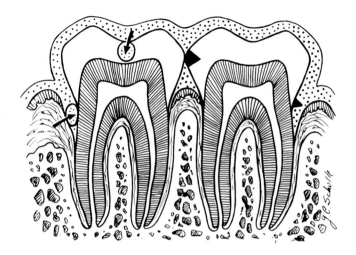

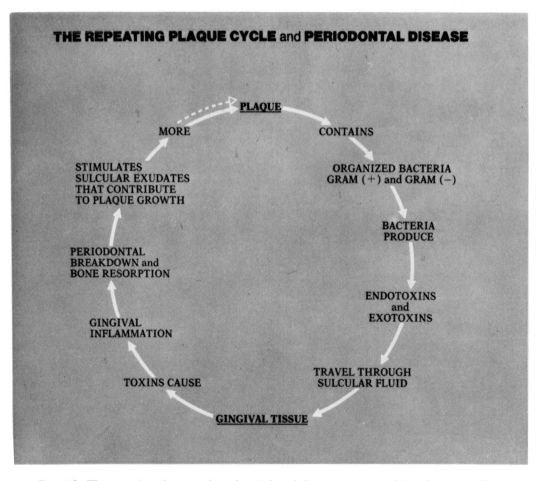

FIG. 4-3. The repeating plaque cycle and periodontal disease (courtesy of Teledyne Aqua Tec).

teria surrounding the teeth and tissues of the oral cavity (Fig. 4-2). Two areas of heavy bacterial accumulation are represented by circles. In these concentrations of organized bacteria, arrows represent nutrients flowing from the oral cavity, furnished by the food eaten by the host, and the serum exudate that is released from the gum tissue to feed the bacterial plaque. Disease is portrayed by the existence of edematous or puffy tissue, the presence of decay between the teeth, the loss of soft tissue and bone, and the formation of calculus. The symptoms represented are the aftermath of an infectious disease. If the cycle is not broken and bacteria are allowed to remain, there is the possibility of further pocket formation and more extensive progression of the disease with the alveolar bone eventually being destroyed (Fig. 4-3).

The mechanism of periodontal disease is more complicated when host resistance is integrated in the system for analysis. It has been known for a long time that the lack of vitamin C produces a disease called scurvy. This affliction causes the gums to bleed, the teeth to become loose and fall out. This sounds very much like the description of periodontal disease. In applying nutrition there is an attempt to reduce the susceptibility to disease and increase the resistance of the host by using what is known to be beneficial. Vitamin C is considered necessary to strengthen the tiny blood vessels of the gums. It is used in the formation of the connective tissue and the periodontal membrane that holds the teeth to the bone. A balance of resistance and susceptibility comes about by considering the total body function instead of just the local environment.

Calculus is not the main irritant, but rather .the bacterial waste products from the living plaque are the cause of periodontal disease. Calculus is the mineralization that occurs within the plaque next to the tooth. It is porous and rough and the bacteria can attach to it. Its formation continues as new plaque becomes old plaque and solidifies and extends itself towards the gum tissue. This further acts to produce stagnant areas away from the flow of saliva and holds the dental plaque close to the gum tissue next to the food supply coming from the gingiva. Calculus is not a totally solid material, and there are bacteria present within the matrix of the calculus itself; however, it is the pooling of the bacteria, waste products, dead tissue cells, and dead bacteria that is the most destructive (Fig. 4-4).

The process of dental disease is multifactorial. All teeth do not decay in the presence of sugar and bacteria and their acids. Approximating surfaces of teeth do not decay equally; bilateral surface areas of decay are sometimes observed, for example, the mesial of the right and left upper molars having decay present similar in location and amount. Tissue is variable in its reaction to the bacterial plaque. Many different possibilities are present that make it more complex as a problem to analyze because of the specific factors that are involved with each patient. What the dentist and his staff are concerned with is studying those components that have a direct bearing on what can be done in controlling dental disease. Further impetus will be gained by those who have the capacity to find the answers when they know that the dental profession is willing and able to apply mea-

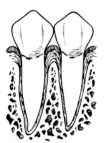 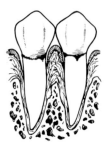 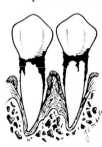

FIG. 4-4. Progression of periodontal disease (adapted from the American Dental Association).

sures that will modify the components that cause disease.

TESTING FOR UNDERSTANDING

It is one thing to conduct procedures; it is another to understand the why of them in their relationship to dental disease. Further understanding of the mechanism of dental disease is possible by observing tests conducted with the patient. Facts at first appear to be separate entities, but as data are obtained they begin to correlate and help form ideas of the processes that combine to make the symptoms and signs that we acknowledge as disease. They are not separate factors that are involved but rather an on-going reaction. By separation of the different elements, the process is evolved that directly relates to the patient and helps us grasp concepts and establish a working knowledge of disease control.

Throughout the control program, testing and evaluation continue, and the disease mechanism progressively becomes more understandable to the patient. It comes as a flow of interesting information instead of a mass of foreign material thrust at him all at once. The facts and hypotheses are given to him at his own rate of acceptance and in a form that is easily assimilated. Tests, handled properly, can have a tremendous motivational impact on the patient and the dental staff as well. Figure 4-5 shows a laboratory test center.

The tests to be discussed will be presented in the order in which they appear on the Test Record (Fig. 4-6) and as they are conducted in the control program referred to in this text. Tests do not contribute to health unless action can be instituted to modify areas of need. It is necessary to put the many tests and data together to form a basis of recommendation. One test alone is not significant. Reliability comes from a broader base of information and cross-checking and analyzing one condition against the other.

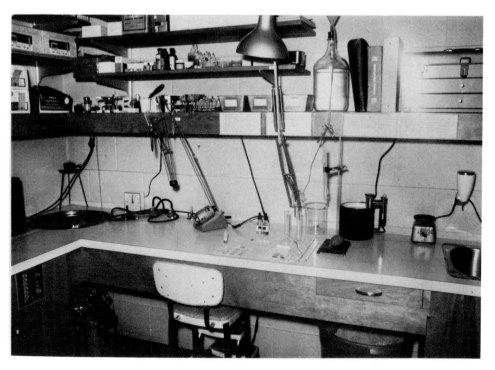

FIG. 4-5. Test Center in a laboratory.

TEST RECORD

Name _____ Date _____ Chart # _____

Phase I
Snyder Test   _____   _____   _____   _____
                 24 hour   48 hour   72 hour   96 hour

Phase II
Lingual Ascorbic Acid Test _____ seconds
Oral Hygiene Evaluation   Excellent - 0   Good - 1   Fair - 2   Poor - 3
Calculus Evaluation   Excellent - 0   Good - 1   Fair - 2   Poor - 3
Number of restored teeth _____   Number of new carious lesions _____

Disease Control # 1
D-K Test (-1 +1   ideal) +2 +3 +4   Oral Hygiene Index past staining _____
Condition of gums: Condition of bone:
  Tender _____   Loss of crest _____
  Bleeding _____   Bone atrophy _____
  Character of tissue _____   Vertical pockets _____
  _____
  Pocket formation _____   Need for water spray _____
Microscopic Observation:
  Few active bacteria _____   Well organized _____
  Well organized with spirochetes _____   Massive bacterial population _____

Disease Control # 3
Salivary Analysis:
  Unstimulated salivary flow _____   average young adult 3.7 ml
  Stimulated salivary flow _____   average young adult 13.8 ml, low 8.0 ml
  Stimulated salivary viscosity_____   seconds (saliva)
                      _____   seconds (water)
              Ratio   _____   = time for 4 ml saliva   Normal 1.3-1.4
                                                time for 4 ml water   High 2+
  Acid Buffering Capacity _____ drops: 14 drops excellent, 10 adequate, 5-6 poor
  Alkaline Phosphatase _____ Bodansky Units: inactive   slightly active
                                                     moderately active   highly active
  Acid Phosphatase _____ Bodansky Units: slightly active   moderately active
                                                    highly active

Disease Control # 5
Oral Glucose Clearance Test _____ minutes

Disease Control # 6
Nutritional Evaluation - Dietronics
Food Groups: Cereal _____ Protein _____ Veg.- Fruit _____ Dairy _____
Daily Calcium _____: Daily Phosphorus _____: Calc/Phos ratio _____

Disease Control # 7   Date _____
Snyder Test # 2   _____   _____   _____   _____
                      24 hour   48 hour   72 hour   96 hour
Fifteen Minute Caries Test _____

Snyder Test # 3   Date _____

_____   _____   _____   _____
 24 hour   48 hour   72 hour   96 hour

FIG. 4-6. Test record.

The Snyder Test

This test is used to determine color-imetrically the metabolic activity (acid production) of Lactobacilli in the saliva. Since fermentable carbohydrates are necessary for the proliferation of these organisms, a carbohydrate medium containing bromcresol green as an indicator is used. The only microorganism other than Lactobacilli that have been found capable of growing in the Snyder medium, which has a pH of 4.8 to 5.1, are Pediococci and some strains of yeast. Pediococci are rarely found in the mouth, and most yeasts are unable to produce enough acid to cause the indicator to change color.

The acid produced by the bacteria changes the color of the medium, and since the rate of color change is proportional to the number of bacteria present in a given volume of medium, it follows, that this is a method of determining the approximate amount of Lactobacilli in a given volume of saliva.

The Snyder test is of value in diet therapy in controlling caries. It can be indicative of the carbohydrate content of a patient's diet since fermentable carbohydrates feed the bacteria. The greater the amount of sugar ingested, the greater the increase in number of these bacteria, which ultimately leads to the greater production of acid.

All procedures that remove plaque and areas where bacteria can stagnate will lower the Lactobacillus count. Before this test is used in diet therapy, all carious lesions should be restored, leaky fillings repaired, and the oral hygiene brought up to the highest possible standards. Food patterns can then be altered and will be reflected by a lower Lactobacillus count. To lower results of the Snyder test in the presence of carious lesions and poor oral hygiene requires a diet so austere that it is not always acceptable to the patient.

Modified Snyder Test

The agar is prepared and used without melting and cooling. The patient drools

sufficient unstimulated (stimulated saliva will lower the count) saliva into a prepared culture tube so that it covers the top of the medium. The culture tube is then incubated at 37° C. for 96 hours. It is read and recorded daily.

The color of the medium changes from blue green (negative) to yellow (positive). This is caused by the acid produced by the Lactobacillus as it penetrates the culture medium. It is read as follows:

No color change — negative

Beginning color change to yellow from top of medium down + or 1+

One half of the medium yellow + + or 2+

Three fourths of the medium yellow + + + or 3+

All of the medium yellow + + + + or 4+[1]

The rapidity of color change indicates the number of bacteria that are present. The greater the change the greater the amount of acid production, which is caused by a large number of microorganisms.

The form in Figure 4-7 is used to record the daily readings of the Snyder test. The results are transposed to the patient's records.

The Snyder test is taken during Phase I of the examination or in Part A of disease control appointment 1 (Chapter 7). This test indicates to the dentist, who communicates it to the patient, the extent of the Lactobacillus involvement in the oral environment prior to treatment. If disease exists, it helps to explain it; if disease does not exist and the test is positive, it indicates the need for preventive measures.

Lingual Ascorbic Acid Test — Pro-C Kit

This test is used to determine the tissue ascorbic acid status in patients. Vitamin C appears to play a significant role in maintaining sound healthy gums and is utilized in the formation of the supporting tissue surrounding the teeth.

This test seems to correlate very well with the patient's needs on a subjective level. Changes in the oral mucosa have been

[1] Courtesy of Dr. Arthur Alban.

SNYDER TESTS

Letter	Recorded	Date	Name	24 hour	36 hour	72 hour	96 hour

FIG. 4-7. Snyder test recording form.

noted after therapeutic doses of vitamin C. Broken blood vessels or petechiae on the palate and bleeding gums have been helped by the taking of vitamin C.

This test is determined by the amount of time (in seconds) that is required for 1 minim of the test solution to decolor when placed on the dorsum of the dried tongue. The interpretation:

Less than 20 seconds: Satisfactory tissue ascorbic acid status

20 to 30 seconds: Marginal tissue ascorbic acid status

Greater than 30 seconds: Poor tissue ascorbic acid status

The Pro-C Kit is listed under Supplies for Testing in Chapter 3.

D-K Caries Activity Test

This test demonstrates the response of microorganisms within the plaque to the addition of sugar. It consists of an acid indicator in a concentrated sucrose solution that turns from yellow to red in the presence of the acid that is produced by the bacteria. The source is listed in Chapter 3.

Sufficient plaque is necessary to conduct the test, and it has been found effective to do this experiment during Part A of disease control visit 1.

Salivary Flow and Viscosity

It is felt by many investigators that the rate of salivary flow and its viscosity are related to caries activity. It appears that the caries rate is greater with deficient salivary flow and that there is less decay with abundant amounts of saliva. Thick, ropy, viscous saliva is associated with more than an average amount of carious lesions while thin saliva of low viscosity is connected with the finding of a relatively few carious lesions. The tests used in determining the salivary flow measure both stimulated and unstimulated saliva collected for a given time.

There can be many causes for decreased saliva, two being emotional and physical. A decrease can be either permanent or temporary. It is felt that some nutritional deficiencies, particularly of nicotinic acid and other members of the vitamin B complex, as well as excessive consumption of refined carbohydrates inhibit the salivary flow. Some drugs such as antihistamines also decrease this flow.

The measurement of salivary viscosity and its ratio to the viscosity of water is determined by the use of the Ostwald pipette.

There is no evidence that the viscosity changes with age. There is considered to be a correlation between viscous saliva and the excessive and frequent consumption of sugar and other refined carbohydrates. Reducing sugar intake may be effective in reducing the viscosity in some patients. The tests for salivary flow and viscosity are a part of Young's Caries Etiology Kit listed under Supplies For Testing in Chapter 3.

The saliva for these tests is collected on visit 3, and test results are related to the patient on visits 5 and 6, at which time they are correlated with the diet.

Acid-Buffering Capacity of Saliva (Modified Dreizen Test)

The ability of saliva to contribute to the buffering capacity of the plaque is an important factor in caries resistance. The capacity is measured by the ability of saliva to resist pH changes upon the addition or formation of acids. A poor buffering capacity is generally associated with rampant caries. An excellent buffering capacity is correlated with teeth relatively free from decay.

The buffering capacity of saliva is related to the bicarbonate buffer system and in all probability to the acid-base equilibrium of the body. The metabolism of fruits and vegetables produces alkaline residues, and patients whose salivary buffering capacity is low often eat few fruits and vegetables. If the patient's food survey indicates that this is true, he should be encouraged to increase the consumption of these foods. This test is also a part of Young's Caries Etiology Kit and is performed and discussed at the same time as the other salivary tests (Fig. 4-8).

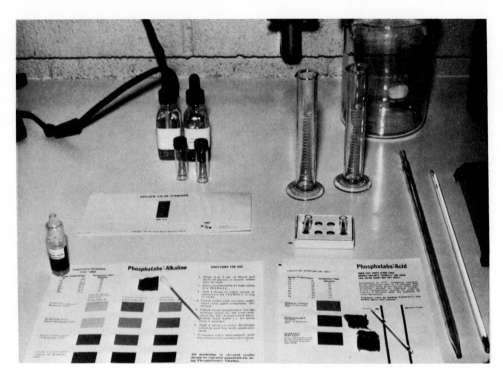

FIG. 4-8. Salivary testing.

Oral Glucose Clearance Test

This test provides information on the ability of a patient's mouth to retain carbohydrate for a given period. It demonstrates through the use of Tes-Tape and a candy bar the oral clearance time for glucose (Fig. 4-9).

Existing evidence is not conclusive, but investigators believe that glucose retention is directly related to caries susceptibility. Long clearance time would indicate that the glucose would feed the bacteria for a longer than desired time. It would be suggested to the patient that he refrain from eating cariogenic foods between meals and that his oral hygiene be of a high standard. This is another test included in Young's Caries Etiology Kit and is conducted during the discussion of cariogenic foods in the disease control program.

Fifteen-Minute Caries Conduciveness Test

This test evaluates the conduciveness of the oral cavity to dental caries. It is based on the rate of activity of reductase enzymes in the saliva. Reductase activity is high in caries-prone mouths and low in nonconducive mouths.

The test consists of mixing together stimulated saliva and a reductase reagent and observing the color change after 15 minutes. It evaluates the adequacy of the oral hygiene techniques and is conducted on the 1-month or visit 7.

The materials to be used for this test are shown in Figure 4-10 and are available through Loyola University School of Dentistry (Chapter 3).

The acid and alkaline phosphatase tests appear on the test record but are not discussed in this text. We are conducting these tests within our private practice to determine their application.

The tests now available are but representatives of an effort to find the answers. More research, more facts, and more statistics will further enable the acceptance of criteria. The dentist himself can take the initiative and test and correlate what appears to be sig-

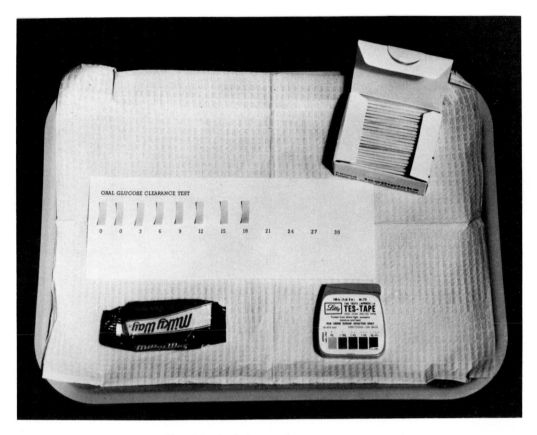

FIG. 4-9. Oral glucose clearance test tray.

nificant. He has the opportunity to directly relate clinical findings and could in this manner raise the present level of understanding of dental disease.

As researchers are able to provide more complete knowledge of the disease process, then the capacity to handle the subject of testing will build further confidence and provide a broader approach that will result in a better selection of control measures.

RELATING THE DISEASE PROCESS TO PATIENTS

The disease process is not discussed with the patient until the patient becomes involved in the control program. Information may be given in answer to specific questions that patients ask, but the understanding of what is happening must be tied in with what the patient can do about it. The two cannot be separated. This will make disease control more meaningful and eliminate the shutting off of the learning process by just giving information before the patient is ready to receive and accept such data. People learn by doing. Having a dentist explain and expect action provides a weakness in patient relationship that cannot be cemented over by any manner of verbal persuasion. The patient must be first genuinely concerned about himself or, if he is a parent, he must be interested in seeing that his child receives the benefits of controlling disease.

It is at the first appointment in the control program that the patient receives an overall background of the prevalence of dental disease. With this, he realizes that fate has not singled him out for this condition. Patients need to be continually reminded that decay and periodontal problems are diseases. This brings to their attention the necessity for understanding and the importance of controlling the known factors that contribute to their problem. It is learning the *why* behind the subject that changes a control program from just going through the motions of doing techniques to one that has a definite concept behind it with purpose. This thorough grasping of the preventive approach leads the way to success because it points out that what is accomplished must be complete and thorough. Brushing the teeth is not sufficient. It is the understanding that the dental plaque must be removed when the teeth are brushed and then acting to make it a fact. The extra effort is small, but the difference it makes is significant to the dental health of the individual.

The Use of Visual Aids

Information can be related to dental patients by audiovisual presentations.

However, a verbal account by the *dentist* establishes a person-to-person relationship that is the basis for developing the motivation and enthusiasm that result from this type of service. A conversational atmosphere is conducted, and an attempt is made to directly relate to the patient and achieve a response between the patient and the dentist.

Visual aids can be helpful in further assisting patients to better understand the disease mechanism, or they can serve as a means of reinforcement to what has been discussed. Some may desire to use films, flip charts, and illustrations drawn on a blackboard or on drawing paper. A clever innovation is the Plackey Cube developed by Dr. Arlen D. Lackey and his wife, Heather (Chapter 3). It is a plastic picture cube depicting the mechanism of disease (Fig. 4-11).

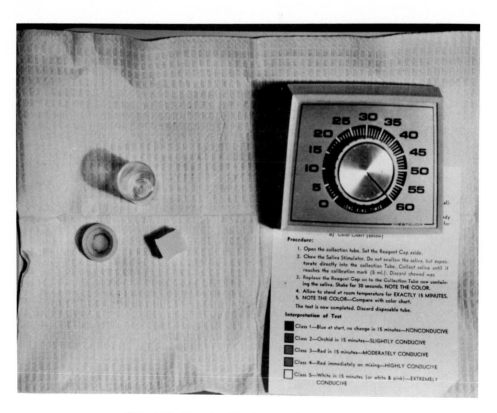

FIG. 4-10. Tray for 15-minute caries test (Rapp).

Visual aids, if properly executed, do help to increase the likelihood of learning and the retention of learning, whereas words alone can be misunderstood. Any device is only an aid and not the sole means to create a background for understanding the forces that must be combated. The use of two or more senses at the same time increases the capacity for learning.

Communicating the Test Results

There is more to preventive dentistry than applying oral hygiene skills. It is also the application and the relation of scientific knowledge to the patient. The tests provide a means to directly relate to the patient the actuality of living organisms in his *own* mouth. The patient can see how food–sugar– enables bacteria to complete their life cycle and produce end products that are destructive to the tooth, the gums, and the jaw bone. He is better able to understand the reasoning behind curtailing these organisms. The results emphasize the importance of the reduction of fermentable carbohydrates and what steps to take to increase the host resistance through nutrition.

The form Personal Dental Profile (see Fig. 6-26) summarizes for the patient the conditions that exist in his mouth prior to treatment, the results of saliva testing, and nutritional factors that relate to food selection. This form is used in discussion with the patient on visit 6 (Chapter 6).

The Use of Dental Knowledge

To understand, appreciate, and follow through, the patient should have some knowledge of dentistry. The dialogue to convey this message is kept short, simple, and uncomplicated. The information is specifically directed at the age level and educational level of the patient and is discussed on visit 4 in the control program (Chapter 8). The topics include:

The structure of the tooth

Use of fluoride, its mechanism and its
   value

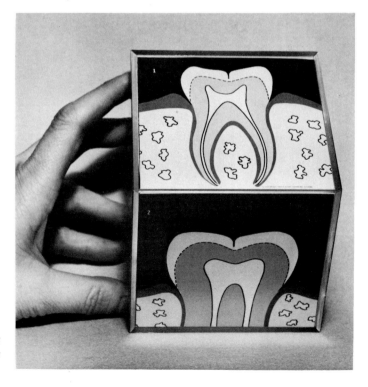

FIG. 4-11. The Plackey Cube (courtesy of Plackey Learning Systems).

Discussion of decay
Review of x-rays, bite-wing x-rays
Abscessed teeth caused by decay
Missing teeth
Areas of decay
Restorations
Areas of bone loss

The patient's chart, x-rays, and diagnostic models are used to communicate the mechanism of dental disease and answer the *why* so he can believe and know that what he is doing is of sound basis. His understanding of the diagnosis makes him better able to appreciate the treatment provided.

5

*The number of cleaning
devices should be few but
effective; the techniques
should be simple but thorough.*

Teaching Guide for Oral Hygiene

THE MECHANICS OF ORAL HYGIENE

The manufacturers of items discussed in this chapter are listed in Chapter 3 under Preventive Inventory.

Disclosants and How to Use Them

Plaque is a term used to describe the little world of bacteria that adheres to the tooth and related structures within the mouth. It is generally colorless in appearance. The disclosing dye is used as a teaching aid in identifying and locating the plaque formation on the teeth and soft tissues.

The staining procedure enables the patient to determine the areas of the mouth that are not being cleaned, and from this measures can be taken to adjust techniques to meet these cleaning requirements. The disclosant serves as a check after the cleaning methods have been mastered and the habit pattern established.

Disclosants are available in tablet, liquid, and swab form. The dye is water soluble and will not permanently stain the teeth or dental restorations. To remove stains from the basins and counter tops, a light bleaching solution or a good liquid detergent can be used. To remove stains from clothing, rinsing immediately and washing in a light bleaching solution are recommended. To remove stains from carpets, a diatomaceous earth compound such as K2r can be applied.

The colors provided by the various disclosants are basic red, blue, and yellow (Plak-Lite). The varying shades of color depend upon the age and the thickness of the plaque — the thicker the plaque the more color it tends to absorb. This causes the mature plaque to appear darker.

The red tablet, often referred to as the pink tablet, is probably the best known of the disclosants; it stains the plaque red. The active ingredient is the dye F.D. and C. red no. 3 (erythrosine). The original flavor was pleasant enough to use but not so palatable that children might eat it as candy. One such tablet, marketed under the brand name Xpose, is fruit flavored.

The liquid disclosants Trace and Plaque-Chek have erythrosine as their active ingredient and color basic red. Trace is a peppermint-flavored solution and Plaque-Chek has a flavor of wild cherry.

Disclosant swabs (Laclede) are available; they color red and are tasteless.

To better enable the patient to distinguish between the bacterial mass and the gingival tissue, a blue dye was developed. This is an important factor as the patient grows older and his eyesight changes. If he is unable to see the pink on his teeth, he will not use the disclosant. The blue color quickly fades from the soft tissues of the mouth. The natural color of the mouth usually has returned by the conclusion of the control visit.

This product is marketed under the name of Dis-plaque and its active ingredients are composed of F.D. and C. approved dyes. This disclosant will stain the plaque in a color range from pink to blue. It has been indicated through study that the blue plaque mass was of greater thickness and more organized than the pink mass. Cocci, rods, and filaments, or combinations, were arranged in parallel rows forming a fan-shaped pattern. The rays were perpendicular to the tooth. The filaments were intertwined to form a meshwork, and spiral organisms and Vibrios were seen. Some mobility was seen in the mass. The pink mass had few organisms, no apparent architecture, and no movement, and no filaments, spiral organisms or vibrios were seen (Block, Lobene, and Derdivanis). This disclosant is available in either tablet or liquid form. It is soluble in water and will not stain restorations.

The practical application in the control program with the two-tone dye system is that the control therapist is able to visualize the areas of the mouth that have been difficult for the patient to adequately clean. The color of the mass is determined by its thickness and therefore indicates its age. Blue is the old thick plaque, pink is the young thin plaque, and purple is somewhere in between. The two-tone system is of special value at the 1-month, 2-month, and recall visits, for these visits are indicative of the technique and habits of the individual patient. It is through these findings that the control therapist is able to evaluate the oral hygiene techniques and teaching methods.

The Plak-Lite is a light that has been developed to view plaque after use of the disclosant containing fluorescein sodium. It stains only the microbial mass yellow, the soft tissue of the oral cavity remaining natural in color. The instrument does not give off ultraviolet light. Its light energy is transmitted in the visible spectrum at approximately 4,600 angstrom units or where dark green appears. The darker the room, the more brilliant yellow the plaque will appear. The mirror on the Plak-Lite is specially filtered, allowing the plaque to be more easily seen; however, a regular mirror can also be used. If there is a large quantity of plaque on the teeth, far greater than average, the plaque will absorb enough disclosant to create a light yellow cast that can be viewed in normal light. It is important that the mouth be rinsed thoroughly to clear the saliva of the solution; otherwise it is difficult to differentiate the plaque. This disclosant is water soluble and is easily removed from clothing with soap and water.

The technique used in disclosing the dental plaque will vary with the type of disclosant used. Since disclosants do color the saliva and the soft tissues, Vaseline is placed on the lips and fingers so the color can be more easily washed off. This is especially important for children because they cannot control the saliva well, and it helps to reduce the staining of cheeks and chins. When the tablet is used, it is chewed slowly and swished with the saliva throughout the mouth to color all the teeth. This requires at least 30 seconds to insure the complete staining of the teeth. The patient is instructed to push his tongue over the surfaces of the teeth. After staining, he should empty his mouth and rinse well with water.

Some patients will not swish the disclosant or color the teeth well. Some are hesitant to view the teeth once they have been disclosed. This is a protective mechanism or a defense set up by the patient to protect himself against the negative information he feels he will receive. Once the patient realizes that he will not be criticized, the problem becomes nonexistent. He will, in fact, remind the control therapist to use the disclosant.

Liquid disclosants can be painted directly on the teeth with a swab or cotton bud. They can also be used by placing 3 to 4 drops under the tongue and then swishing throughout the mouth. A rinse solution can be made

FIG. 5-1. Teeth appearing normal before the use of the disclosant (courtesy of the University of Oregon Dental School).

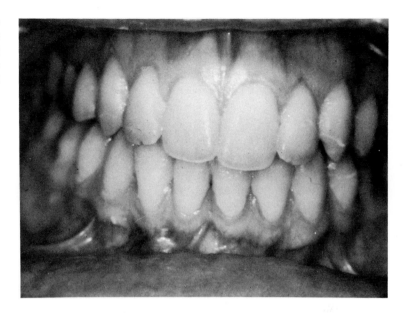

by using 10 to 12 drops per 1 tablespoon of water in a paper cup. When a swab is used it can be moistened slightly either in water or in the patient's saliva and painted on the teeth.

Colored pictures depicting the use of disclosants reinforce in the patient's mind the presence of the bacterial mass in relationship to his brushing technique. The pictures chosen should demonstrate the disclosant used in the control program because that is how the patient sees it in his own mouth. The Procter and Gamble Tablet Test depicts Before Tablet Test, After Tablet Test, and After Brushing Properly and is an excellent selection of colored pictures showing the use of the red disclosant. Pacemaker has a series of pictures illustrating the use of Dis-plaque, the blue disclosant. Figures 5-1 and 5-2 show teeth before and after use of a disclosant.

Dental Floss and How to Use It

Dental floss is a tool used to disorganize and remove the microbial masses that are located below the gum margins and between the teeth on the mesial and distal surfaces.

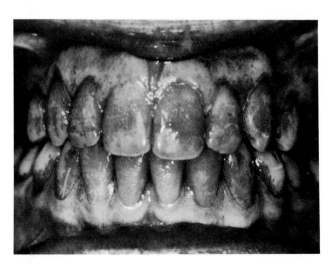

FIG. 5-2. Bacterial plaque after staining by the disclosant (courtesy of the University of Oregon Dental School).

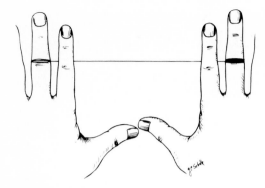

FIG. 5-3. The floss wrapped around the fingers ready for use.

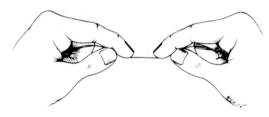

FIG. 5-4. Positioning the fingers on the floss.

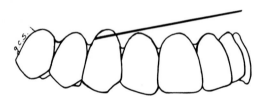

FIG. 5-5. The floss carried into the gingival sulcus.

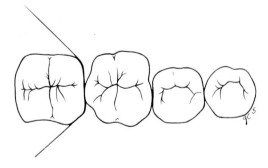

FIG. 5-6. The floss wrapped tightly around the tooth.

There are two types of floss, the waxed and the unwaxed. The waxed floss coats the enamel surfaces of the tooth and is inadequate for removing plaque. It is not recommended for cleaning purposes. The unwaxed floss made to the specifications set forth by Dr. C. C. Bass is designed for easy and effective use. The thin nylon fibers of this floss serve as individual knives or cutting edges as it is manipulated to scrape the plaque from the tooth. This floss spreads easily over the tooth surface, which allows it to be easily passed between the contact points of the teeth.

To clean the tooth adequately, the floss must be carried down under the gum margin until resistance is met, wrapped around the curvature of the tooth, and then scraped upward for its entire length. The fingers used in this procedure are not important. Each patient will develop a technique that is comfortable for himself. There are a few suggestions that are helpful.

The piece of floss to be used should be from 18 to 24 inches long. Most of the floss is wrapped on one finger of one hand, depending upon whether the patient is right- or left-handed and personal preference. (Right-handed persons seem to prefer to wrap most of the floss on a finger on the right hand.) The floss is anchored on a finger on the opposite hand (Fig. 5-3).

As the floss becomes used and frayed, it is scrolled from the finger containing the greater amount to the finger containing the lesser amount. It is important to change the floss at regular intervals in this manner because as it becomes used and frayed it becomes ineffective as a cleaner and will in time break. Occasionally a piece of floss will lodge between the teeth. This usually can be removed by inserting another piece of unwaxed floss or if necessary a piece of waxed floss. If the floss becomes snagged by an obstruction on the tooth surface and cannot be removed, the floss is disengaged from one finger and pulled through to one side.

For better control, more effective cleaning, and less gagging, the fingers should be from 1/2 to 1 inch apart, depending on the size of the fingers (Fig. 5-4). In order to carry the floss deep into the sulcus area the fingers should be on top of the floss as it is taken down into the gingival tissues.

It may be necessary to gently work the floss back and forth to pass between the contact points of the teeth. The floss is kept close to the tooth, and is carried beneath the margin of the gums until resistance is met (Fig. 5-5). The floss is then wrapped around the tooth (Fig 5-6). With the floss held tightly against the tooth, it is cleaned with a scraping up-and-down motion. This can also be accomplished in a single stroke if the fingers have adequate strength.

To clean the distal surfaces of the tooth, both fingers are brought forward toward the front of the mouth. To clean the mesial surface of the tooth, both fingers are pushed to the back of the mouth.

The tooth is clean when a squeaky sound is heard. A diet high in carbohydrate will give the feel of thickness and stickiness as the tooth is scraped because of the bacterial response to the diet.

Each tooth should be cleaned individually. It is best not to cross over from one tooth to the other. The floss can be deep under the gingival tissue and there is a danger of cutting the tissue, and the incisal third of the contact area of the tooth will not be adequately cleaned.

Beginning on the lower back, the fingers are on top of the floss as it is carried down under the gingival margins (Fig. 5-7). As the center teeth are reached the hands are reversed; the hand that was on the lingual or tongue side is now on the facial or cheek side (Fig. 5-8). When the upper arch is flossed, the floss is pushed up using the two thumbs, a thumb and finger, or two fingers (Fig. 5-9).

Floss Threaders. The floss threader is a means by which floss can be carried under fixed bridges, between splinted teeth (5-10), and under low solder joints to remove plaque

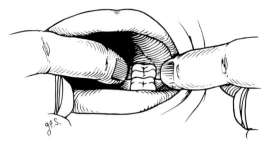

FIG. 5-7. Placement of the fingers on the floss in cleaning the lower left back molars.

and food debris. These are generally made of a pliable plastic or wire.

A length of unwaxed floss approximately 24 inches long is placed through the eye of the threader. The threader is passed through between the abutment (natural) tooth and the pontic (artificial tooth) (Fig. 5-11). Care should be taken not to injure the gum. The threader is then disengaged from the floss.

The floss is manipulated with the index fingers. It is curved toward the tooth as it is carried to below the gum margin of the abutment tooth. With firm pressure, the abutment tooth is scraped in an up-and-down motion until the tooth no longer feels slimy or sticky. The floss is moved to a position under the pontic and scraped in a

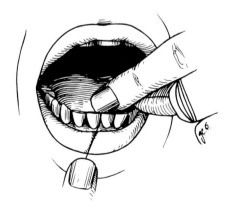

FIG 5-8. The finger positions are reversed as the teeth are flossed from left to right. The floss is to be carried deep on the lingual or tongue side.

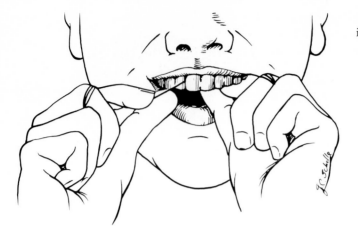

FIG. 5-9. Position of the thumbs in flossing the upper anterior teeth.

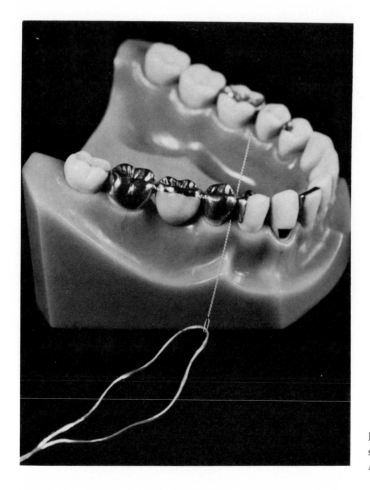

FIG. 5-10. Placement of the E Z Flex floss threader between splinted teeth (courtesy of Tri Arc Productions).

FIG. 5-11. Placement of floss under a bridge using the EEZ-Thru floss threader (courtesy of John O. Butler Co.).

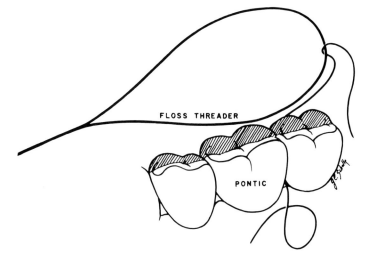

FIG. 5-12. Cleaning under a bridge (adapted from a drawing by Tri Arc Productions).

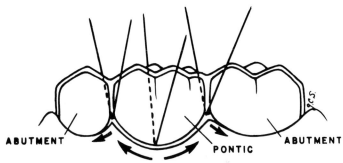

FIG. 5-13. The Floss Aid (courtesy of Floss Aid Co.).

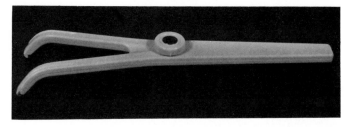

back-and-forth motion (Fig. 5-12). The remaining abutment tooth is cleaned in the manner previously described.

Factors to be considered in selecting the proper floss threader:

1. The threader must be narrow enough to pass between the teeth.
2. The size of the eye must be large enough so that it can be easily seen and threaded.
3. The threader should be long and firm enough to be easily picked up by the fingers after it has been passed between the teeth.

Floss Holders. These instruments can be helpful to the handicapped, to those who have a strong gag reflex, to those who, because of their age or physical condition, are unable to manipulate the floss, and to those who emotionally cannot floss without assistance. They can be used by the mother for the very young child, 2 to 5 years of age. Some children aged 5 to 7 years can adequately floss their teeth by using a floss holder. (*Caution:* The floss holder can become a crutch and serve as an excuse to not floss when it is misplaced or broken. Each child using a holder will in time need

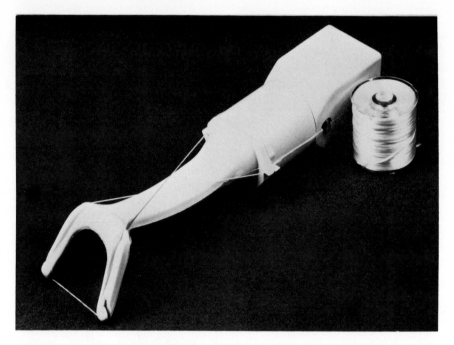

FIG. 5-14. The Floss-Span (courtesy of Texell Products Co. A Rimel photo, Houston Tex.).

to be taught to use his fingers.) (Fig. 5-13)

One end of a piece of floss approximately 15 inches long is wrapped around the disc, extended up and over the ends of the two prongs, and returned to the disc where it is tightly secured. To insure tautness, the prongs can be forced together, but no closer than 3/4 inch.

The cleaning of the tooth is accomplished in the same manner as when the fingers are used. To clean the distal surfaces of the tooth, the Floss Aid is pulled (curved) forward and the tooth is scraped with an up-and-down motion. The mesial surface of the tooth is cleaned in the same manner except that the Floss-Aid is pushed towards the back of the mouth.

The Floss-Span is another one of several aids that are available. The manipulation of these holders is the same as with the Floss-Aid (Fig. 5-14).

The Toothbrush and How to Use It

The value of the toothbrush is dependent upon the ability of the patient to use it properly. Just "brushing the teeth" will not clean them adequately enough to prevent decay or gum disease.

The toothbrush referred to in the procedures in this text is one in which the bristles when placed into the sulcus will not cause damage to the gingival tissue. It is preferred that the head of the brush contain two rows of bristles (Fig. 5-15), that these bristles be soft, made of nylon, measure .007 inch in diameter, and have ends that have been rounded and polished (Fig. 5-16).

The purpose of a toothbrushing technique is to remove the bacterial mass from the buccal (cheek side), lingual (tongue side), and the occlusal (biting) surfaces as well as the sulcus (under the gum) area of the tooth.

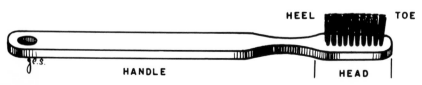

HEEL   TOE

HANDLE   HEAD

FIG. 5-15. The two-row sulcular toothbrush.

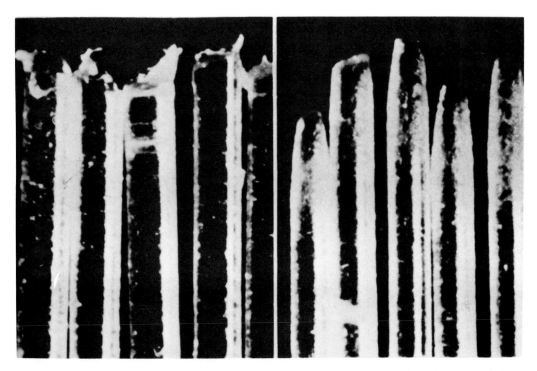

FIG. 5-16. Bristles. Left, ordinary nylon filament. Right, the bristles have been rounded, tapered, and satinized (courtesy of John O. Butler Co.).

The correct way *to hold the toothbrush* is shown in Figures 5-17 and 5-18.

To properly place the toothbrush bristle, it should be directed into the area where the tooth meets the gum (sulcus) at about a 45-degree angle (Fig. 5-19). This is referred to as sulcular brushing.

To help the patient develop a systematic approach to brushing the teeth, it should be suggested to the patient that he begin the procedure on the lower left back molar. The majority of the patients will gladly accept this suggestion, and it becomes their

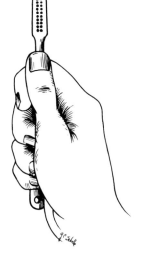

FIG. 5-17. Holding the toothbrush.

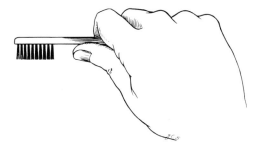

FIG. 5-18. Holding the toothbrush.

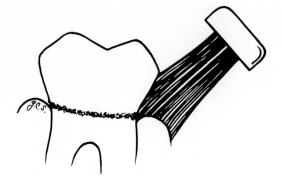

FIG. 5-19. Placement of the toothbrush bristles into the sulcus at a 45-degree angle to the tooth.

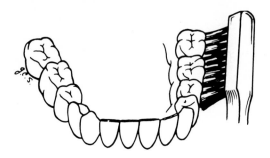

FIG. 5-20. Placement of the toothbrush on the lower left posterior, cheek side.

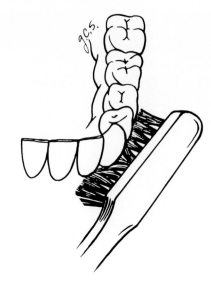

FIG. 5-21. Placement of the toothbrush on the lower left corner, cheek side.

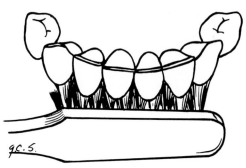

FIG. 5-22. Placement of the toothbrush on the lower anteriors, cheek side.

habit. Others who may be more noncon-forming, more creative, or even more belligerent in nature will establish their own pattern. This is not important. What is important is that they always start in the same place and follow a set pattern. This trains the hand. The patient does not have to think about where he has cleaned and where he has yet to clean. This results in rapid, thorough cleaning. *A systematic approach helps the patient establish the habit.*

To clean the teeth, begin on the left lower arch, the buccal (cheek side) of the last back molar (Fig. 5-20). Keeping the bristles off the occlusal (biting) surfaces, direct them into the sulcus at a 45-degree angle. While maintaining light pressure, vibrate the bristles, using a back-and-forth motion and taking care that the bristles remain in the sulcus. After this area is cleaned, pick up the toothbrush and replace it in the next position. Close the mouth slightly, allowing

the cheek to relax to provide more room for the toothbrush. Proceed from left to right. The number of teeth to be cleaned at one time depends upon the size of the teeth, the size of the jaw, and the size of the toothbrush.

Because of limited wrist action special attention must be given to the corners of the arch as the direction of the toothbrush is changed (Fig. 5-21). Right-handed persons may skip the right corner, and left-handed persons may skip the left corner of the arch.

In the lower anterior (front) region, blanching of the gingival tissues will be noted when the bristles are properly placed (Fig. 5-22). The blood is pushed from the tissues as

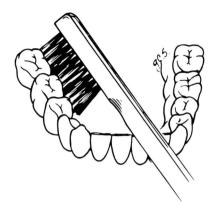

FIG. 5-23. Placement of the toothbrush on the lower right posterior, tongue side.

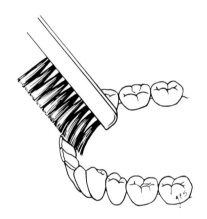

FIG. 5-24. Placement of the toothbrush on the lower anteriors, tongue side.

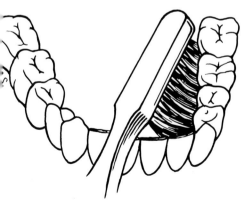

FIG. 5-25. Placement of the toothbrush on the lower left posterior, tongue side.

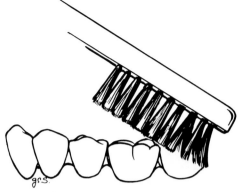

FIG. 5-26. Placement of the toothbrush on the back lower left molar.

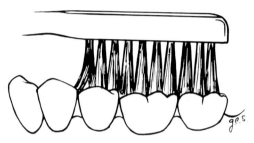

FIG. 5-27. Placement of the toothbrush on the lower left arch, chewing surface.

pressure is applied; as pressure is released the blood returns to the tissues.

To clean the lingual (tongue side), begin on the right last molar, directing the bristles into the sulcus at a 45-degree angle (Fig. 5-23). Proceed from right to left.

To clean the lower anterior teeth, use a short up-and-down motion with the mouth opened wide and the handle of the toothbrush raised sharply (Fig. 5-24). The handle may nearly touch the upper anterior teeth. Clean the first and second bicuspid area. (Fig. 5-25). Proceed to complete the lingual areas.

To clean the occlusal surface of the tooth, begin on the left side. Close the mouth slightly and lift the handle of the toothbrush, allowing a few bristles from the toe of the toothbrush to enter the sulcus behind the last molar (Fig. 5-26).

The remaining occlusal surfaces are cleaned with a short back-and-forth motion. The handle of the toothbrush should be parallel to the occlusal surface (Fig. 5-27).

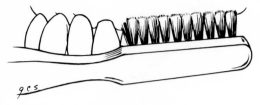

FIG. 5-28. Placement of the toothbrush on the upper left posterior, cheek side.

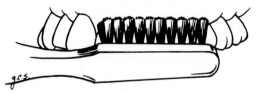

FIG. 5-29. Placement of the toothbrush on the upper left bicuspid area, cheek side.

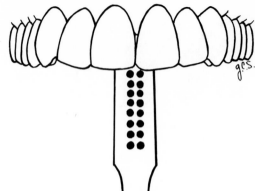

FIG. 5-31. Position of the toothbrush for the upper anterior teeth on the tongue side.

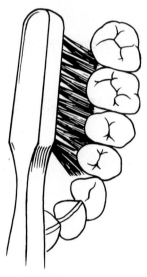

FIG. 5-30. Placement of the toothbrush for the upper right posterior, tongue side.

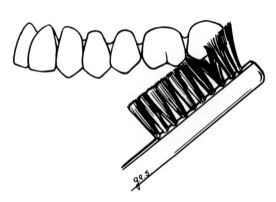

FIG. 5-32. Placement of the toothbrush on the upper left back molar.

Do not forget to clean the incisal (biting) surface of the anterior teeth.

Return to the buccal of the right back molar, and with the mouth slightly closed and using short back-and-forth strokes, clean the incisal two thirds of the tooth to "make it shine." A vertical up-and-down stroke may be used on the anterior teeth that have deep grooves and on crooked or misplaced teeth. Special attention should be given to the corners. Caution the patient not to apply heavy pressure on the toothbrush.

The make-them-shine stroke is familiar for most patients. It resembles their old method of brushing. Children's eyes light up and they smile. Adults give a sigh of relief. It allows the patient time to relax, and he seems emotionally better able to accept the fact that the brushing he has done in the past has been incorrect. By returning to this stroke his self has been preserved, he has been doing a part of it right.

This completes the cleaning of the lower arch. After mastering the technique, the patient will not return to these teeth again. It is a completed task, well done, with no part of the tooth being forgotten. One half

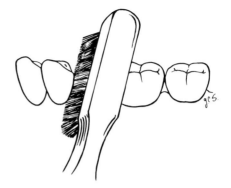

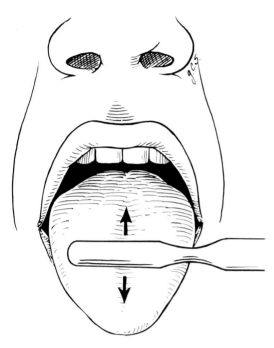

FIG. 5-34. Placement of the toothbrush in cleaning the area of a missing tooth.

FIG. 5-33. Brushing the tongue.

of the short-range goal of brushing the teeth has been accomplished. The patient now prepares to clean the upper arch.

The teeth on the upper arch are cleaned in the same manner as the teeth on the lower arch except in reverse. Begin on the left buccal (cheek side) of the last back molar (Fig. 5-28). With the mouth slightly closed, direct the bristles at a 45-degree angle into the sulcus, and using light pressure, vibrate the bristles with a back-and-forth motion, taking care that the bristles remain within the sulcus. Proceed from left to right (Fig. 5-29), giving special attention to the corners as the direction of the toothbrush is changed. The blanching of the gingival tissues of the anterior (front) teeth indicates that the bristles of the toothbrush are properly placed into the sulcus.

To clean the lingual (tongue side) beginning on the right side, properly align the toothbrush by placing the head parallel to the arch with the handle touching the first "front" tooth on this, the right side. Then direct the bristles into the sulcus at a 45-degree angle (Fig. 5-30). Proceed from right

to left. The lingual of the anterior teeth is cleaned with an up-and-down motion, using a few bristles from the toe of the toothbrush. The handle of the toothbrush is lowered sharply straight down (Fig. 5-31).

To clean the occlusal (biting) surface, begin on the left side. The mouth is opened wide, the handle of the toothbrush is lowered downward, and a few bristles are directed into the sulcus behind the last back molar (Fig. 5-32).

Do not forget to clean the incisal (biting) surface of the anterior teeth. As in the lower arch, the incisal two thirds of the teeth are cleaned with a general back-and-forth motion, unless conditions (crooked and misplaced teeth, deep grooves) warrant a vertical up-and-down motion, to "shine" the teeth.

The final step in the cleaning of the mouth is to brush the tongue. Begin at the tip of the tongue and gradually work towards the back (Fig. 5-33). The stroke used is a matter of personal preference, usually a posterior-to-anterior stroke is used on small tongues and a circular motion on large tongues. Brushing the tongue does improve its health for it increases the circulation and removes the bacteria and waste products that can cause bad breath. There will be an occasional patient who has been told by a mother or grandmother to brush his tongue, but the control therapist should be prepared for a bewildered response from the patient.

One technique will not clean all teeth in all mouths. The technique to be used is dependent upon the size, shape, and position of the teeth, the size of the mouth, and the presence or absence of the gag reflex.

Suggestions for troublesome areas:

Areas of missing teeth: The distal of the tooth can be cleaned by angling the toothbrush so that the bristles can be directed into the sulcus (Fig. 5-34). It may also be treated as if it were the last tooth in the arch.

The lingual of the first and second bicuspids can be cleaned by handling the toothbrush as a pencil and directing a few bristles from the toe of the brush into the sulcus. The toothbrush handle should be upward and out from the corner of the mouth. The lingual of the back molars can be cleaned in the same manner. If a four-row bristle brush is used, the lingual of the back molars can be cleaned by placing the toothbrush with the bristles split and allowing a few to enter into the sulcus with the majority of the brush up and over the occlusal surface of the tooth. The buccal surface can be cleaned in the same manner.

Crooked or misplaced teeth may have to be cleaned individually rather than as a part of a unit of several teeth.

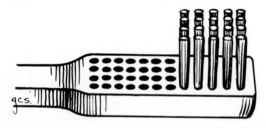

FIG. 5-35. Modification of the toothbrush to enable cleaning hard to reach areas such as the lower anteriors on the tongue side.

Bristles can be cut off from the heel of the toothbrush (Fig. 5-35). This can be used on the lingual of the anterior teeth.

The *Proxabrush* (Fig. 5-36) consists of a handle that holds interchangeable brushes of varying sizes. It is designed to clean between the teeth and inaccessible areas. It is effective for plaque removal in healthy mouths as well as in those with periodontal involvement. The patient should be cautioned to occasionally check the end of the brush and see if the wire is exposed as the bristles are worn. The handle can also be used to hold the rounded toothpick.

The toothpick is used to remove the bacterial mass from areas inaccessible to the toothbrush bristle. It can be used to clean around tipped, crooked, or misplaced teeth, along the lingual surface of the back molars, and the buccal surface of the third molar. It is effective in disrupting the plaque in periodontal pockets and in cleaning the root surfaces of the teeth. It is also used to clean areas where bleeding continues to occur 4 to 5 days into the control program. It should not be used to remove food from between the teeth, as is commonly done, for it can cause injury if it is placed wrong and jabbed into the gingival tissue.

Several handles that hold the rounded toothpick are available. The most common are the Proxabrush handle, which also holds various size core brushes, and the Perio-Aids #1, 2 & 3.

The *Perio-Aid* #1 is a plastic holder with tapered holes at either end. A rounded toothpick is inserted into one of the holes and the excess broken off. The toothpick is moistened with tap water. This softens the wood and allows it to swell, holding it firmly in place. Perio-Aids #2 and #3 are plastic

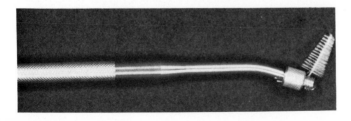

FIG. 5-36. The Proxabrush (courtesy of John O. Butler Co.).

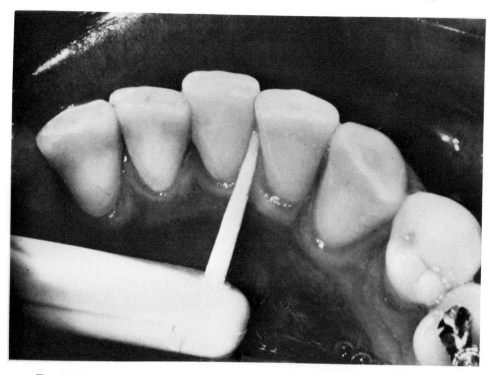

FIG. 5-37. Placement of the Perio-Aid #1 (courtesy of Marquis Dental Mfg. Co.).

handles with adjustable screw ends. The World's Fair brand of toothpick is recommended by the manufacturer for use in the Perio-Aid.

The Perio-Aid is held by the fingers in a pencil-like grip with the little finger braced on the chin. The toothpick is used by directing the end of the toothpick at right angles to the tooth (Fig. 5-37, 5-38) and scraping back and forth three or four times to remove the plaque. The difficult and inaccessible areas are generally along the gum line on the lingual side. The toothpick can also be used as a brush by removing the tip and splitting the end. It is recommended that this not be chewed or broken by the use of the teeth.

To remove the toothpick from the Perio-Aid, it is pressed on a hard surface in reverse of the loading direction. If it is too wet, it should be allowed to dry before further attempts are made to remove it.

The *rubber tip* located on the handle of some toothbrushes is used for further stimulation of the gums. Stimulator handles are also available separately. The base of the rubber tip is placed between the teeth with the tip pointed toward the occlusal surface (Fig. 5-39). It is held at a 45-degree angle to the gum. Pressure is maintained against the gum, and the tip is vibrated.

Oral Irrigation and Technique

Rinsing the Mouth. The purpose of rinsing the mouth is to remove the material that has been loosened with the floss and the toothbrush bristle. The teeth and the mouth are rinsed by forcing water vigorously back and forth through the teeth several times.

A saline solution (½ teaspoonful of salt to 1 cup of warm water) may be desirable for patients with tender gums. This solution is soothing and healing to the gums and provides a means for the patient himself to make the gums feel better.

The Oral Irrigator. The primary purpose of water irrigation is to cleanse the pockets that form along the side of the root of the

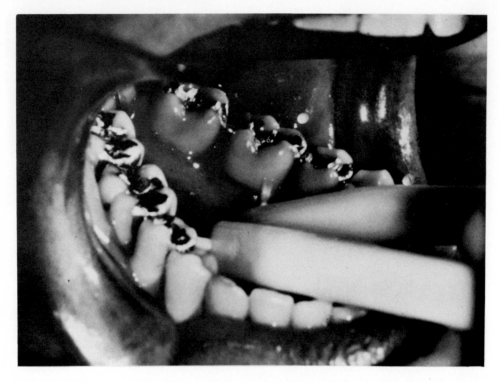

FIG. 5-38. Placement of the Perio-Aid #1 in cleaning along the gum line of the lower posterior on the tongue side (courtesy of Marquis Dental Mfg. Co.).

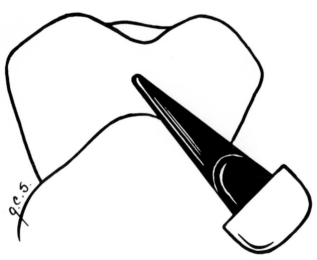

FIG. 5-39. Placement of the rubber tip.

Fig. 5-40. The Dento-Spray (courtesy of Texell Products Co.).

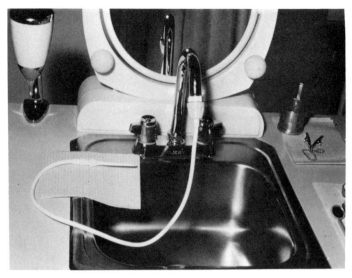

tooth. The flushing action of the water removes the serums discharged by the sub-gingival tissue that feeds the microcosm as well as the related toxic material that accumulates within these pockets. In addition to this, the irrigator is used to remove already loosened plaque formation and food debris from around and under fixed bridges and orthodontic appliances.

The water used should be warm and the flow gentle. Heat dilates the blood vessels and stimulates the activity of the tissue cells. It assists the normal reactionary processes occurring in inflammation and stimulates

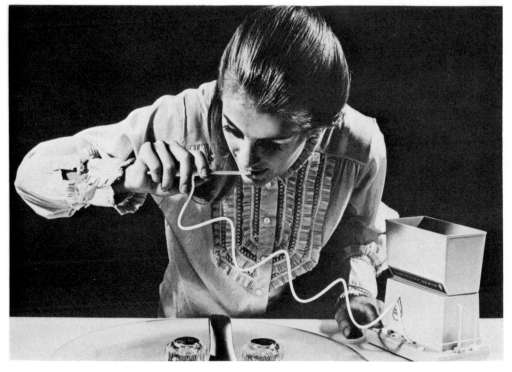

Fig. 5-41. Correct position of the arm in using the Water Pik water spray (courtesy of Teledyne Aqua Tec).

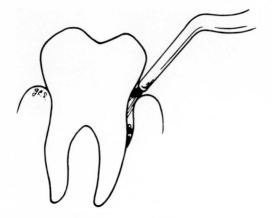

FIG. 5-42. Placement of the tip and direction of water irrigation when using a continuous flow water spray.

tissue repair and healing. The force of the water that is directed toward the subgingival tissue must be gentle. In the healthy state, this tissue can easily be damaged. In the diseased state, the epithelial lining of the sulcus tissue is absent or is in a weakened condition and is an inadequate barrier to prevent the bacteria and other foreign substances from entering into the tissue. The value of any irrigation is related to the quantity of the microbial material remaining after the procedure has been completed.

Oral irrigators are available in faucet and electric pump sprays and in continuous water flow and pulsating or intermittent water action.

The faucet continuous water–flow irrigators are Dento-Spray (Fig. 5-40), POH Oral Water Spray, and Hydro Water Toothpick. These maintain a continual flushing action into the desired areas.

A Technique. The water temperature and pressure should be adjusted before the procedure is begun. The water should be warm, not hot. The pressure should be enough to remove loosened material, but not enough to cause discomfort in the mouth. The patient leans over the sink and raises the elbow so the arm will be horizontal to prevent water from running down the hand and arm (Fig. 5-41). The angled tip of the irrigator allows the patient to direct the flow of water along the tooth surfaces and into the subgingival spaces. The lips should be slightly closed but opened enough to allow the water to run freely from the mouth into

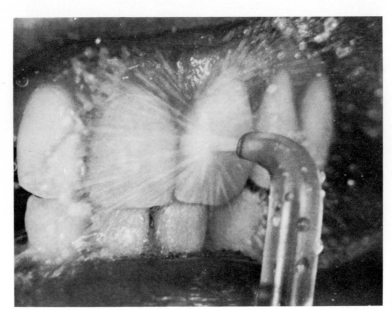

FIG. 5-43. Placement of the tip when using the Water Pik (courtesy of Teledyne Aqua Tec).

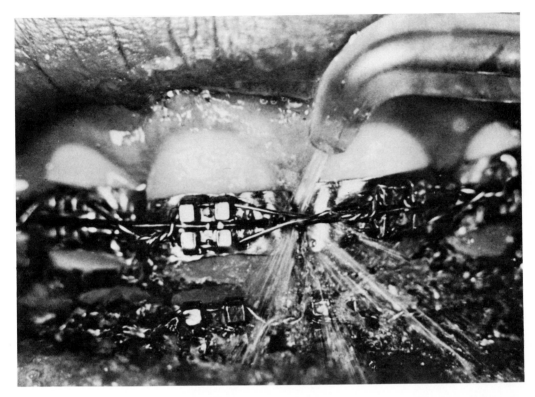

FIG. 5-44. Use of the Water Pik in cleaning orthodontic appliances (courtesy of Teledyne Aqua Tec).

the sink. The water should not be allowed to accumulate in the mouth.

The tip is directed towards and almost touching the gum line into the periodontal pockets (Fig. 5-42) or around and under fixed bridges and orthodontic appliances. The force must be gentle but adequate enough to remove loosened particles.

The pulsating or intermittent water action devices are available in faucet (Pulsar) and electric pump (Water Pik) irrigators. In the pulsating action, the jet of water is directed at a 90-degree angle to the tooth surface close to the gingiva (Fig. 5-43). From there it enters into the subgingival sulcus where the blood is forced from the capillaries at the point of impingement, or where the water strikes the tissue. At the interval between, the tissue contracts, expelling the water and its contents from the subgingival sulcus. The

capillaries refill with blood. This creates a massaging and pumping action that contributes to the healing process. For undamaged gingival tissue, the pulsed water jet with pressures up to 90 psi may be acceptable. For inflamed tissue, water jet pressures of between 50 and 70 psi are recommended.

All irrigators are used similarly by beginning at the back of the last molar and slowly progressing along the buccal and lingual surfaces of both the upper and the lower arches. The procedure is completed by rinsing the chewing surfaces of the teeth as well as the other areas of the mouth. The user must avoid directing the water stream under the tongue.

Water irrigation is a valuable aid to the orthodontic patient in caring for his mouth during treatment (Fig. 5-44). Control measures should be completed before the place-

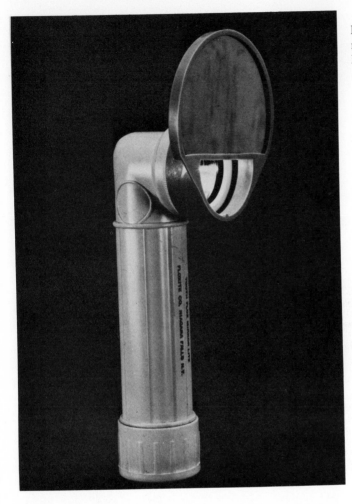

FIG. 5-45. Tooth Flox Mirror Lite, a magnifying mirror attachment for 2-inch flashlight (courtesy Floxite Co. A Jenkins photo).

ment of bands, after which the best possible oral hygiene techniques should be continued, which would include the thorough rinsing of the oral cavity.

Several types of water irrigators are desirable in the control room for demonstration purposes. Most patients have heard of water sprays, but they do not know how to use them or why they are beneficial. If both faucet and tank types are available for discussion, the patient may compare and be better able to select the one to meet his needs. The dentist may have a recommendation not only for the need but also for the type that would be advantageous to the patient.

Illuminating the Mouth

Lighting is important in the beginning appointments of the control program. It will seem to the control therapist that the tooth appears as a foreign object to the patient. In the past it has been something that he should brush and the dentist should fix. The patient will learn to floss his teeth without the mirror if *he* so desires, and it would seem that it is his choice to make. Few persons know the shape, size, or placement of their teeth. A mirror aids in the placement of the floss during this learning period.

Those with good hand-to-eye coordination can often floss faster using a mirror. Patients who have not developed this ability will automatically look away from the mirror as they use the floss.

The patient will learn to know the feeling of the bacterial mass on his teeth by the use of his tongue, but he should know by viewing, unless his eyesight does not permit it,

FIG. 5-46. Floxite mirror-lamp set (courtesy of Floxite Co. — a Jenkins photo).

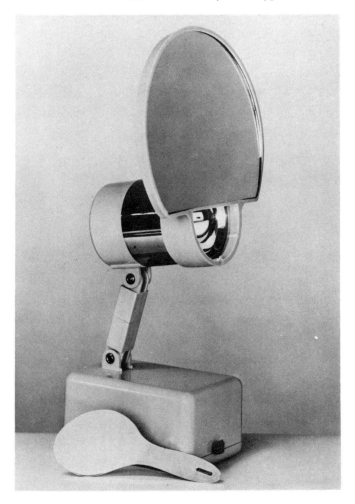

the pattern that the bacteria form on his teeth. Certain areas that are hard for him to clean can only be detected by having available suitable lighting and an adequate mirror.

The makeup mirror, which can be obtained in several price ranges, often will provide sufficient light both at home and in the office. The flashlight, an item nearly every household has, is perhaps the least expensive and the most effective. Mirror attachments are available to make the flashlight even more effective. The magnifying mirror fits a 2-inch flashlight such as the scout type (Fig. 5-45). The mirror focuses up to 4 inches from the mouth.

The mirror-lamp can be set on the table top or fastened to the wall (Fig. 5-46). It is powered with a 7-volt current transformed from 115 AC. Its 5-inch magnifying mirror focuses up to 7 inches from the mouth.

In addition to these aids, plastic magnifying mirrors can be used to reflect light into the lingual and hidden areas of the teeth and gums. The magnifying mirror attachment for flashlights, the mirror-lamp set, and the detail reflectors are available individually or in sets. Plastic mouth mirrors can be useful for home care and are inexpensive. Penlight flashlights with a mirror attached such as the Oral-Lite are available (Fig. 5-47).

The Use of Toothpaste

The teeth can be cleaned with or without the use of toothpaste. Dental disease can be controlled by the use of water in the brushing procedure. Patients are accustomed to the use of toothpaste. It does help

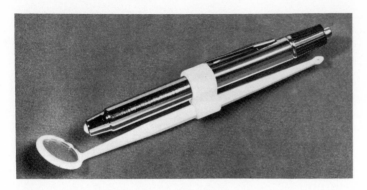

FIG. 5-47. Oral-Lite (courtesy of Professional Budget Plan).

to clean and polish the teeth, is flavored and sudsy. If toothpaste is used, it should contain fluoride to gain the beneficial effect that it has on the enamel surface of the tooth and any inhibitory effect that it might have on the bacterial plaque itself.

THE AIDS USED IN PRESENTING ORAL HYGIENE

Models of the Teeth

To assist in demonstrating the techniques of flossing and brushing, commercial models of the complete dentition, upper and lower arch (Fig. 5-48) and the patient's diagnostic models are used.

Models are available with removable teeth. They are used to demonstrate the flossing technique by passing the floss under the area representing the gum tissue. Models with removable teeth help to duplicate the patient's own mouth (in case of missing teeth) when diagnostic models are not available. Technique models of dental restorations that include fixed bridges and other restorative dentistry are of value in demonstrating specific cleaning procedures.

The patient's diagnostic model (Fig. 5-49) is an invaluable awareness tool. It allows the control therapist to determine the best approach in cleaning, and it shows the

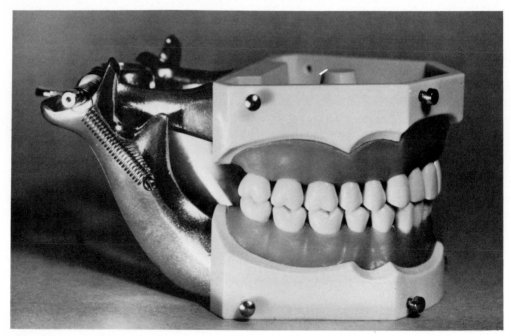

FIG. 5-48. Demonstration models (courtesy of Columbia Dentoform Corp.).

FIG. 5-49. Patient's diagnostic models.

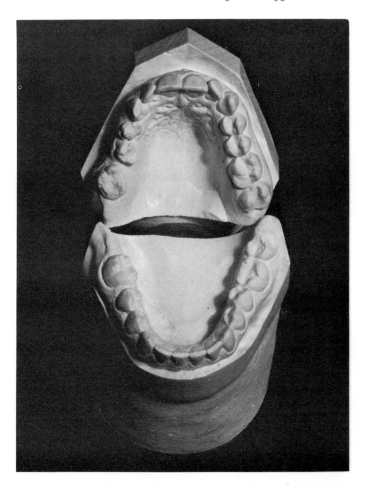

patient what his mouth is really like. He can see the crooked teeth, and those that are misplaced or missing. He becomes more aware of the "holes" caused by decay. He realizes that something should be done, and he begins to think about placing a higher priority on his dental needs.

Take-Home Information

The pamphlet *Research Explores Plaque* (Fig. 5-50) is used to preview the material that will be presented in the control program as well as to provide authority for the program to follow. This pamphlet is well written and easy to read. It is divided into three sections — the problem of plaque, the control of plaque, and progress through research.

The specific home instructions are printed on the dentist's prescription form (Fig. 5-51).

This indicates that the information comes directly from the dentist and is approved by him. People are familiar with prescriptions and are conditioned to follow their directions. The supplies that the patient will be required to provide once the program is completed are listed as home supplies.

The Personal Oral Hygiene Instruction Sheet (Figs. 5-52, 5-53) provides written instructions in the techniques of using the disclosant, brushing the teeth, flossing the teeth, and rinsing the mouth, as well as general information concerning the tissue response, schedule to follow, and frequency of cleaning.

The order of procedure in learning the thorough cleaning techniques may seem detailed and confusing to the patient. For this reason the home care schedule (Figs. 5-54 to 5-56) is given to the patient at the appropri-

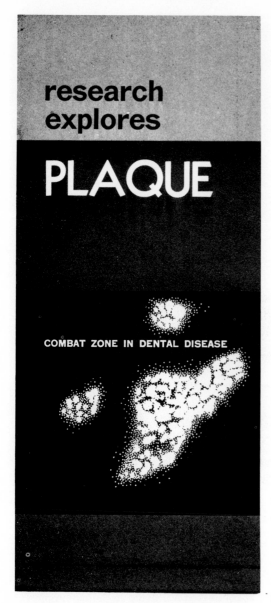

research explores

PLAQUE

COMBAT ZONE IN DENTAL DISEASE

FIG. 5-50. Pamphlet Research Explores Plaque (courtesy of National Institute of Dental Research).

ate time within the control program: week 1, floss the teeth, stain the teeth, and brush the teeth; week 2, floss, brush, and then stain to determine the areas that are difficult to reach; and week 3, floss and brush. Adults stain once a month to check the technique. Children stain once a week.

Flossing is done before brushing so that

the patient will be conditioned to include it in the routine of brushing the teeth. Most people come into a dental office with their habit of brushing their teeth already established. The difficulty does not lie in learning the proper use of the toothbrush and dental floss, it lies in doing it. *The habit of flossing must be established.* Flossing before brushing enables the patient to feel with his tongue what he has cleaned. Brushing prior to flossing will clean a large area of the tooth surface; the mouth will feel better because of the plaque removal and because of oral stimulation. So the patient reasons, "Why not skip flossing tonight? I am very tired, it is late, I'll do it tomorrow." Tomorrow never comes, and flossing is dropped from the cleaning procedure.

The teeth are stained after flossing rather than before because one of the best indicators of the condition of the gums is the presence or absence of bleeding. If the gums are pink, it may be difficult to determine the amount of bleeding. The disclosant will also color the fingers. If several days elapse between visits, specific instructions should be given to the patient (Fig. 5-57).

The pamphlet *A New Plan to Keep Your Teeth for a Lifetime* (Fig. 5-58) discusses the merits of a clean tooth and illustrates the flossing and brushing technique. It also depicts before and after the use of the disclosant.

This pamphlet or similar printed material provides authority to the methods presented to the patient. The illustrations can be related to the patient's mouth. Pictures in the sequence presented in the Tablet Test show the patient what his teeth looked like at his first visit. The "after" picture is what his teeth look like after he has cleaned them. The patient knows this is true; he can *feel* it as well as see it in his own mouth.

The pamphlet *What You Need to Know and Do to Prevent Dental Caries (Tooth Decay) and Periodontal Disease (Pyorrhea)* (Fig. 5-59) discusses several cases and the results that were achieved through adequate oral hygiene. The research that this pamphlet was based upon was conducted at the

FIG. 5-51. A list of supplies needed by the patient to carry out the procedures.

ARTHUR GARY DINGERSON, D.D.S.
513 NORTH MORRISON ROAD
VANCOUVER, WASHINGTON 98664

BNDD AD1007524
REG. No. 7141

TELEPHONE 694-5211

NAME_____ AGE_____

ADDRESS_____ DATE_____

℞   HOME SUPPLIES
Toothbrushes: Butler #210 - 2 row or #411 - 4 row
Pycopay for Gum Care Brush
POH Brush
Oral B Sulcus

Unwaxed dental floss: Butler, POH, Prevent a Tape

Disclosing tablet or liquid - any brand

FIG. 5-52. Personal Oral Hygiene Sheet Instruction (courtesy of POH).

PERSONAL ORAL HYGIENE INSTRUCTION SHEET

TO SHOW BACTERIAL COLONIES

Place a disclosing wafer in your mouth and slowly dissolve. Push the wafer around the teeth with your tongue to bring the wafer in contact with the front, sides and insides of all your teeth.

INSPECTION

Using a well lighted mirror examine your mouth. The bright red areas are the living bacteria.

BRUSHING

The most important areas to be cleaned with the toothbrush are (a) the biting surfaces in the pits and grooves, (b) the sides of the teeth and, (c) the space between the gums and the teeth. Brush the stained material away with short strokes, applying the tips of the bristles to the area with light pressure, and moving the brush back and forth with a vibrating or circular motion. This type of brushing will dislodge the soft stained material by the digging action of the ends of the bristles wherever they can be applied. Flaring of the bristles indicates too much pressure is being used.

FLOSSING

Cut off a piece of floss about 2 feet long. Wrap one end around the right index for the purpose of anchoring or holding. Use the right thumb to hold the floss against the right index finger. Grasp the floss with the left hand so that the length of floss, about one inch long, is between the hands. The following illustrations show how to hold the floss in the different areas of the mouth.

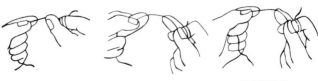

UPPER RIGHT TEETH   UPPER LEFT TEETH   ALL LOWER TEETH

Slip the floss between each pair of teeth by drawing it gently and slightly back and forth. Carry the floss under the gum until you feel definite resistance without discomfort, and then scrape it up along the sides of both teeth.

RINSING

After cleaning all the teeth with dental floss, rinse your mouth by forcing water vigorously back and forth between the teeth in order to remove material that has been loosened or dislodged but not removed by the floss.

REINSPECTION

After brushing and flossing your teeth, re-examine them carefully. Any red stained areas remaining should be removed. It is not possible to remove absolutely all of the adherent stained material. The important thing is to reduce its thickness appreciably. By morning, all traces of the stain will be gone from the mouth.

FIG. 5-53. Personal Oral Hygiene Sheet Instruction (courtesy of POH).

GENERAL INFORMATION

Before retiring is the most important time for cleaning the teeth and the proper time for staining and thorough P.O.H. The important thing is to be sure you remove the new growth of bacteria.

Your gums may bleed slightly and become tender during your first two weeks on P.O.H. This soon ceases and the previously inflamed tissue rapidly heals. No bleeding or discomfort will be experienced from any reasonable manipulations of the brush or floss in the future.

Stain your teeth every night for the first week, then clean the teeth to remove the stain. The second week, clean your teeth first and then stain them to see if you missed any area. After you learn the correct personal hygiene method the stain will no longer be necessary for daily use. Use it to check yourself once a week from then on.

THE MEASURE OF SUCCESS

The bacteria grow back every 24 hours. By using the stain solution you know where they grow and live. You must remove them thoroughly, systematically, and effectively daily or the bacteria will accumulate in such large number that disease results.

NO ONE CAN DO IT FOR YOU
THE SUCCESS OF THIS TREATMENT
RESTS SOLELY IN YOUR HANDS

ARTHUR GARY DINGERSON, D.D.S.
513 NORTH MORRISON ROAD
VANCOUVER, WASHINGTON 98664

TELEPHONE 694-5211

BNDD AD1007524
REG. NO. 7141

NAME_____ AGE_____

ADDRESS_____ DATE_____

R̶ This week # 1
    Floss your teeth
    Stain your teeth
    Brush your teeth

    Tonight, brush the food off
    Do not brush into the gums

    Tomorrow, do not clean your teeth
    before your appointment.

FIG. 5-54. Oral hygiene instructions for week 1 of the control program.

FIG. 5-55. Oral hygiene instructions for week 2 of the control program.

ARTHUR GARY DINGERSON, D.D.S.
513 NORTH MORRISON ROAD
VANCOUVER, WASHINGTON 98664

TELEPHONE 694-5211

BNDD AD1007524
REG. NO. 7141

NAME_____ AGE_____

ADDRESS_____ DATE_____

℞   This week # 2
      Floss your teeth
      Brush your teeth
      Stain your teeth

    Establish a habit
      Clean at the same time each day
      Floss first; then brush
      Always start at the same place
      Follow a set pattern

FIG. 5-56. Oral hygiene instructions for week 3 of the control program.

ARTHUR GARY DINGERSON, D.D.S.
513 NORTH MORRISON ROAD
VANCOUVER, WASHINGTON 98664

TELEPHONE 694-5211

BNDD AD1007524
REG. NO. 7141

NAME_____ AGE_____

ADDRESS_____ DATE_____

℞   This week # 3 and thereafter
      Floss your teeth
      Brush your teeth
      Stain your teeth once a week

                  month

    TO CHECK YOUR TECHNIQUE

FIG. 5-57. Specific oral hygiene instructions.

ARTHUR GARY DINGERSON, D.D.S.
513 NORTH MORRISON ROAD
VANCOUVER, WASHINGTON 98664

TELEPHONE 694-5211

BNDD AD1007524
REG. NO. 7141

NAME_____ AGE_____

ADDRESS_____ DATE_____

℞

      Saturday - - - - - Floss
        Sunday   Stain
                  Brush

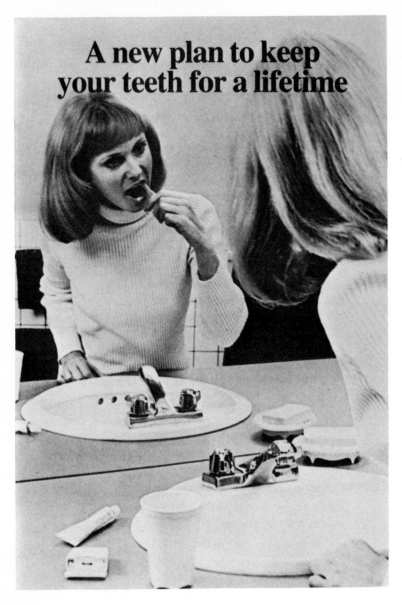

A new plan to keep your teeth for a lifetime

FIG. 5-58. A pamphlet discussing the oral hygiene that provides the opportunity to keep teeth for a lifetime (courtesy of Procter & Gamble Co.).

University of Texas Dental Branch at Houston by Dr. Sumter Arnim.

SUMMARY

The tools and the techniques used to control dental disease may seem complicated and time consuming. It does take the average adult about 2 weeks to master them, after which the teeth can be adequately cleaned in less than 5 minutes.

The written material is important in that it repeats the story again through words and pictures and emphasizes that which is obtainable.

FIG. 5-59. A pamphlet discussing cases and results achieved through oral hygiene (courtesy of Dr. Sumter Arnim, the Journal of the North Carolina Dental Society, and the Dental Health Division, North Carolina State Board of Health).

WHAT YOU NEED TO KNOW AND DO

TO

PREVENT DENTAL CARIES (Tooth Decay)

AND

PERIODONTAL DISEASE (Pyorrhea)

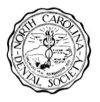

Reprinted from the Journal of the North Carolina Dental Society,
Volume 46, No. 4, August 1963 by the Division of Dental Health,
North Carolina State Board of Health in cooperation with the North
Carolina Dental Society.

6 | *The relationship of food intake to dental disease needs to be defined and then followed by an approach that is knowledgeable and workable.*

Relating Nutrition to Dental Disease

WHY NUTRITIONAL COUNSELING IN A CONTROL PROGRAM?

Nutrition plays a vital role in the control of dental disease. One purpose of nutritional counseling in the dental office is to inform and help the patient eliminate those foods that are implicated as obstacles to dental health. The decay of the teeth from acid-producing bacteria can virtually be eliminated through the restriction of refined carbohydrates in the diet.

More important and certainly of far more reaching and lasting effect is to attack dental disease by increasing the resistance and decreasing the susceptibility of the host through proper nutrition. This is done by having the patient become involved in analyzing his nutritional needs or deficiencies, or both, and improving his food selection so that he will provide himself with sufficient nutrients (vitamins, minerals, fats, carbohydrates, protein, and water).

Application of diet improvement comes about through the motivation acquired by the patient. The dental health team's real contribution is to provide information and facts that can be converted into action. When the patient can actually experience the difference that adequate nutrition contributes, then self-motivation will take place.

WHO SHOULD DO THE NUTRITIONAL COUNSELING?

The person who will be most effective in assisting the patient in nutritional counseling will be the one who, having established rapport with the patient, has presented a helpful attitude and has previously contributed to achieving worthwhile results. This is the control therapist who, in the appointments leading to this discussion of nutrition, has set the stage to make it a worthwhile experience. The control therapist more than any other member of the staff knows and understands the patient. Both patient and counselor have come to respect and trust each other and have become friends. Without this prior conditioning it is doubtful whether a true exchange or communication can take place that has any meaning. It takes time, energy, and devotion to build to a point where personal eating habits can be the topic of conversation.

It is to the advantage of the person filling this role as counselor to have had some training in nutrition and to have applied and analyzed its results in the home laboratory—a family. Budget buying, food handling, meal planning and preparation, plus the problem solving that evolves around the family eating habits all contribute to a better understanding of what is involved. The unmarried person without this experience or training in nutrition will need to spend more time in preparation.

Nutritional information is not difficult, and any competent person can be as successful as a person who is professionally trained in the field. The counselor, however, must

100

know from personal experience what it is to feel good because of her own selection of food and eating pattern. She should not expect of her patient what she herself does not do.

WHO SHOULD RECEIVE NUTRITIONAL COUNSELING?

All patients—child and adult—should receive advice concerning nutrition. The young child often becomes exposed to the deleterious food habits of the baby sitter, his friend across the street, or his relatives. A diet history may reveal a situation such as the one of a 4-year-old boy with ten surfaces of decay in the primary teeth because of his daily stay with a baby sitter during the preceding 3 years. Candy, cookies, and Kool-Aid have pacified him and the other children in her care.

Another example is the teenager whose first cavities appeared the year she went away to school. The reason given was that there was no fluoride in the drinking water, but could it have been the lack of mother's supervision in the foods that were eaten? Still another is the teenager who selects his own breakfast which consists of cinnamon rolls and pop at the high school cafeteria.

Discussion may reveal the young mother of two children, aged 1 and 4 years, who is chronically tired and irritable and who constantly screams at the children. Throughout the day she drinks coffee and eats doughnuts and provides the children with cookies and Kool-Aid.

Another to be helped is the adult in his 40s whose teeth are loosening and beginning to "fall out" because of the lack of bone to support them, or the grandfather who is thin, irritable, and tired and is failing rapidly.

These are but a representation of the various age groups that will present themselves for control of dental disease and of the different states of health encountered in the individuals receiving nutritional counseling. The number of decayed, missing, or filled teeth should not be the criterion for providing nutritional counseling. To present nutritional counseling only when active decay is occurring is "control" dentistry. The lack of active caries may indicate the lack of sugar in the diet, but it does not indicate adequate nutrition. The thin emaciated child with no cavities can be eating very few sugar foods, very little nutritious food, and more than adequate amounts of "junk" food containing empty calories. Inadequate nutrition is not found in any one section of the country or in any one economic class of people or in any one age group. It is found next door, across the street, or down the block. It can be found among one's own family, friends, and relatives.

Food selection and eating patterns are influenced by cultural, religious, and economic factors as well as social pressures, but what seems to be a major contributing factor to widespread nutritional inadequacies is the lack of knowledge. People want to feel good, and those patients who are prepared to receive and are motivated to respond to nutritional counseling are gaining great benefits from such a program. It so happens that what is good for the teeth, bone, blood vessels, and soft tissue of the mouth is also of value for the rest of the body and vice versa. The body is not segmented into a dental section and a medical section but is one unit. Nutritional counseling must take into consideration the total person, including his life style.

Patients want to know the role that food plays in decay. Food supplies a basic need of the human body, and patients want to know what foods should be eaten, what vitamins and minerals are, and why they work in the body. People desire a better life for themselves and their family, and adequate nutrients play a major role in supporting and maintaining this life.

Food selection and eating patterns are passed down in families from one generation to another, and in some families they are not easily disrupted. Change will not occur unless there is a recognition of a need for change. In some families it is easy; the patient will return home and announce to the family that changes are to be made and so it is done. This may throw the family unit into chaos for a while, but as the months and years pass the dental bills dwindle into nothing, the general health of the family noticeably improves, and emotional stability returns. With other patients the change will be slow but with definite progress. Not until the need for a balanced diet takes precedence over other needs will some patients change their eating habits. Eventually this may occur for those without this awareness, and they too may reap the benefits that adequate nutrition provides.

WHEN SHOULD NUTRITIONAL COUNSELING BE INSTITUTED?

Nutritional counseling is conducted on visits 5 and 6 of the program. By this time the patient has become quite adept at accomplishing the oral hygiene techniques and rapport has been established between the patient and the control therapist.

The food histories, the 5-day Food Diary and Dietronics, to be discussed later, are initiated on the first visit of the disease control program. This allows enough time to elapse for the completion of the analysis of the food histories as well as the preparation of the patient for counseling.

NUTRIENTS AND WHY WE NEED THEM

The information given to the patient concerning nutrients and their functions in the body should be simple. He is interested in the nutrients that his body requires and which foods contain them. The information should be related to him in a manner that he can accept or he will not take action. What the patient really wants to know is how it affects him and his family.

The material that follows in this section is a discussion of the nutrients that are considered in the control program. Questions arise that require drawing upon basic knowledge about the different nutrients and how they function. Each nutrient is discussed in the order in which it appears on the Dietronics printout.

Proteins

Proteins are made up of twenty-two amino acids, eight of which cannot be synthesized by the body and therefore must be obtained from the food we eat. These eight are known as essential amino acids and they must be replenished daily. Protein is one of the most important nutrients used in the body. Proteins are used for building, development, maintenance, and repair. There are indications that diets supplemented with protein improve the gingival state, improve the depth of the sulcus, and decrease the mobility of the tooth (Clark, Cheraskin, and Ringsdorf). Proteins are also components of the enzyme and endocrine systems.

Protein in foods is divided into two groupings. Complete protein is found in animal sources—egg, milk, cheese, fish, chicken, beef, and pork—and contains the eight essential amino acids. (Note, however, that gelatin, a food from an animal source, is an incomplete protein.) Incomplete protein found in plant foods—grains, nuts, fruits, and vegetables—is missing or deficient in one or more of the essential amino acids.

The combining of foods containing complete proteins from animal sources with those containing the incomplete proteins of plant food allows the body to utilize the protein more effectively, providing the two complement each other with the missing component. This combination must be eaten at the same meal because the amino acids are not stored for any great length of time.

High protein diets can be tolerated by healthy individuals. Excessive protein is used for energy. A high protein diet could be hazardous for people with liver or kidney disease.

Calories

A calorie is a measure of energy needed by the body to transform food energy to body energy. The number of calories required by an individual is dependent on several factors:

Body size: Larger allowances than those

indicated for the reference man or woman are indicated for a larger body size and smaller allowances for a more diminutive size.

Age: Because of lessened physical activity and a decrease in metabolic rate, the energy requirements usually decline after early adulthood. This depends upon the activity level of the individuals.

Activity: The greater the energy expended, the greater the caloric requirement. There is evidence that persons consume more calories than they need.

Climate: A temperature range of 68° F. to 77° F. applies to most living conditions in the United States. Slightly more calories are needed for those living in colder climates because of the extra clothing they carry. If the body is inadequately clothed body cooling occurs, and caloric needs increase because of the increased metabolic rate associated with shivering and other related body movements. More calories are required for persons working in high temperatures (98° F. to 100° F.) because of the increase in the metabolic rate as well as in body activity to maintain thermal balance.

Pregnancy: Energy requirements are increased because of the building of new tissue in the placenta and the fetus and because of other related activities during pregnancy.

Lactation: The energy requirement during this period is proportional to the quantity of milk produced.

The calorie requirement for infants, children, and adolescents should be interpreted with caution because of their physical activity.

(A test for obesity: A person may be overweight if more than one inch of skin and underlying tissue can be placed between the fingers on the side of the chest.)

Carbohydrates

Carbohydrates in food are sugars, starches, and cellulose. Simple carbohydrates include the monosaccharide and disaccharide sugars. Complex carbohydrates are the polysaccharides (starches) and cellulose.

Monosaccharides are:

Glucose, also known as dextrose, whose source is grape sugar and corn sugar, is contained in such foods as honey, fruits, and corn syrup.

Fructose, fruit sugar, is the sweetest and is found in honey, fruits, and corn syrup.

Galactose is the sugar found in milk.

Sorbitol and *mannitol* are alcohol derivatives from glucose and mannose. Sorbitol is used as a sweetening agent in diabetic food. It has little effect on the blood sugar because it is slowly absorbed from the intestine.

Disaccharides, or sugars consisting of two monosaccharides, are:

Sucrose, cane sugar, beet sugar, and maple sugar, is available as a highly refined pure carbohydrate—white sugar.

Lactose, milk sugar, is the only carbohydrate of animal origin that is significantly nutritious.

Maltose is formed through a process of malting barley.

Polysaccharides are:

Starch, the most familiar polysaccharide, is a natural product made by plants for energy. It is stored in the stems, seeds, roots, and tubers. Food sources are potatoes, and corn and other whole-kernel grains.

Glycogen, or animal starch, is stored in the liver and muscle.

Cellulose:

Cellulose constitutes the framework of plants. It is not digested by man and so serves as a food source of roughage and bulk.

The major function of carbohydrates is to provide energy. Glucose is the major energy source for the central nervous system. It facilitates the oxidation of fats. If sufficient carbohydrate is not available, protein will be used as an energy source. If a meal provides more glucose than the liver or muscle can store, it will be turned into and stored as fat. Sucrose and glucose supplements have been shown to increase plaque formation, worsen the gingival state, increase the sulcus depth, and increase tooth mobility.

Vitamin A

Vitamin A keeps the skin and mucous membranes healthy. It helps resist infection and is essential for growth and vision. Vitamin A deficiency can lead to night blindness, a condition in which it is difficult for the eyes to see in the darkness after having been adjusted to bright lights.

Protein malnutrition will result in poor intestinal absorption as well as impairment of the transportation of vitamin A in the bloodstream. Laxatives, antibiotics, and some other drugs, as well as some diseases related to its malabsorption, will decrease absorption of vitamin A from the intestinal tract.

Vitamin A is fat soluble; therefore it is not easily absorbed except in the presence of fat. It is stored in the liver. Foods of animal origin provide the only immediate source of vitamin A. Green and yellow vegetables contain a substance called carotene that is changed in the body to vitamin A.

Foods high in vitamin A are carrots, green leafy vegetables such as turnip greens, beet greens, mustard greens, spinach, kale, chard, and broccoli, butter, whole milk, liver, and fish.

Vitamin E

Vitamin E is composed of seven forms, which are called tocopherols. One of the most common forms, alpha tocopherol, is the most active in the animal and human body. Most researchers consider alpha tocopherol synonymous with vitamin E.

Functions of vitamin E include its utilization as an antioxidant and a conserver of oxygen. It reduces the need for oxygen because the cells perform more efficiently. Vitamin E is a vasodilator and anti-coagulant, and it hastens wound healing and tends to prevent scars.

The requirements for vitamin E increase as the intake of polyunsaturates increases in the diet. Polyunsaturated fats are easily oxidizable, and sufficient vitamin E prevents the destruction of the polyunsaturated fatty acids. Vitamin E is fat soluble, and it must have fat to be absorbed by the body.

Foods high in vitamin E are margarine, salad dressing oil, vegetable oils, eggs, whole-grain cereals and wheat germ oil.

Vitamin B$_1$ (Thiamine)

Vitamin B$_1$ is one of the vitamin B complex. It is involved with the metabolism of fats and carbohydrates. Vitamin B$_1$ and niacin requirements increase with the caloric intake. It is essential for growth, good appetite, digestion, and healthy nerves. Signs and symptoms of its deficiency are poor appetite, nervousness, and irritability. Extreme deficiency can lead to the nervous disease, beriberi. This vitamin is water soluble, and the amount that is stored in the body is negligible.

Foods high in thiamine are liver, pork, yeast, organ meats, whole grains, bread, wheat germ, and peanuts.

Vitamin B$_2$ (Riboflavin)

Vitamin B$_2$ is another of the B complex group and is essential for growth and for good vision. It is used in the metabolism of carbohydrates, fats, and protein. Deficiencies are characterized by burning or sandy eyes that are particularly sensitive to light, nasolabial seborrhea, and angular lesions of the lobes of the ears. (These manifestations can also be due to deficiencies of other vitamins of the vitamin B complex group.) Riboflavin is water soluble and is not readily stored in the body.

Foods high in vitamin B$_2$ are eggs, liver, yeast, milk, whole grains, bread, and wheat germ.

Niacin (Nicotinic Acid)

Niacin is also a member of the vitamin B complex group. It is more stable than vitamin B$_1$ or vitamin B$_2$. Deficiencies can occur in protein-poor diets (the body can convert the amino acid tryptophan into niacin), in chronic alcoholism, intestinal disturbances, pregnancy, lactation, hyperthyroidism, and infections. The deficiency disease of niacin is pellagra, which is characterized by dermatitis, diarrhea, and dementia.

Foods high in niacin are yeast, liver, wheat bran, peanuts, and bran.

Vitamin B₆ (Pyridoxine)

Vitamin B_6 or pyridoxine is a term used to describe a group of naturally occurring pyridines that are interrelated. It is also included in the B complex group and assists in the metabolism of protein as well as in the utilization of carbohydrates and fats. The requirement for this vitamin may increase with the increase of protein in the diet. The signs and symptoms of deficiency of vitamin B_6 are similar to those of B_1 and B_2: cheilosis, stomatitis, glossitis, seborrheic dermatitis, and erythema in the nasolabial folds.

Foods high in pyridoxine are wheat germ, kidney, liver, and other organ meats, ham, legumes, and peanuts.

Pantothenic Acid

Pantothenic acid is still another of the vitamin B complex group. It was discovered in 1939. It is easily destroyed by heat. The calcium form, calcium pantothenate, is soluble in water, more stable in heat, and is generally available. It is used by the body during times of stress.

Deficiency of this vitamin results in a loss of antibody production in animals and man. Signs and symptoms include fatigue, headache, malaise, nausea, abdominal stress, paresthesia of hands and feet, and cramping of the leg muscles.

Foods high in pantothenic acid are liver, organ meats, eggs, yeast, wheat bran, legumes, and cereals.

Vitamin B₁₂ (Cyanocobalamin)

Vitamin B_{12} consists of several related compounds. It is a member of the vitamin B complex group and a by-product in the manufacture of streptomycin. Vitamin B_{12} is essential for the normal functioning of all cells, particularly bone marrow, the nervous system, and the gastrointestinal tract. Lack of it will cause pernicious anemia. Signs and symptoms are sore mouth and tongue, menstrual disturbances, nervous symptoms such as neuritic pain, stiffness in the spine, and difficulty in walking.

Foods high in vitamin B_{12} are liver, organ meats, oysters, salmon, eggs, and beef.

Vitamin C (Ascorbic Acid)

Vitamin C is essential for tissue health. It is necessary for growth and maintenance of teeth, bones, tissues, and blood. It makes the material that cements the cells together, makes walls of blood vessels firm, helps to resist infection, helps prevent fatigue, and helps in the healing of wounds and broken bones.

Vitamin C is water soluble. It is stored in the body, but for only short periods, and therefore must be replenished daily. Heat and air destroy vitamin C.

Some foods that contain vitamin C are citrus fruits, berries, broccoli, tomatoes, green leafy vegetables, baked potatoes, and turnips.

Water-soluble vitamins are lost with the use of alcohol and diuretics such as coffee.

Calcium

Calcium is the substance found in blackboard chalk. The bone and teeth contain 99 per cent of the total body calcium. The remaining 1 per cent is found in the body fluids, soft tissues, and the blood. Calcium provides strength to the bone and teeth. It contributes to muscle contraction, relaxes the nerve tissue, helps blood clotting, and reduces nerve irritability. The way in which calcium is used in the body is determined by the presence of phosphorus and vitamin D.

Foods containing calcium are cheese, milk, bread, nuts, dried figs, dried beans, dried peas, dark green leafy vegetables, dandelion greens, mustard and turnip greens, collards, kale, and broccoli.

Phosphorus

Phosphorus provides teeth and bone with rigidity. The bones and the teeth contain

70 to 80 per cent of the total body phosphorus with 20 to 30 per cent being stored in the soft tissues. Phosphorus is used in the quick release of energy in muscular contractions. It is concerned with protein synthesis and cell production. It also assists in the transportation and absorption of other nutrients.

Foods high in phosphorus are soya flour, whole wheat, oatmeal, peas, brown rice, whole corn, lima beans, and nuts.

The Council on Nutrition, National Academy of Sciences recommends that 800 mg. of calcium and 800 mg. of phosphorus daily, or a 1:1 ratio, be standard. The balance of calcium and phosphorus may very well have an influence on decay and periodontal disease. A proper balance, that is, a 1:1 ratio, in the relationship of these two nutrients appears to be the soundest approach at the present time.

Magnesium

Magnesium is an activator of many enzymes. Foods high in magnesium are soya flour, whole wheat, oatmeal, peas, brown rice, whole corn, beans, and nuts.

Iron

Iron combines with copper to form hemoglobin. Hemoglobin carries O_2 (oxygen) from the lungs to the tissues and carbon dioxide from the tissues to the lungs.

The human body does not absorb iron very well. Amino acids and vitamin C assist in its absorption. It is presumed that men and boys normally eating enough calories each day receive sufficient iron in the diet. Infants and menstruating females usually do not get enough iron and their diets should be supplemented.

Foods high in iron are liver, organ meats, eggs, dried beans, green leafy vegetables, and oysters.

NUTRIENTS—HOW MUCH DO WE NEED AND HOW DO WE SELECT THEM?

The amount of nutrients required is highly individualized. The state of physical and emotional health, dietary pattern, the age, sex, type of work, and climate all play a role in the amount required by any given person.

Recommended Dietary Allowances

Beginning in the early 1930s, the U.S. Government initiated studies of population groups to determine some minimal quantities of nutrients necessary for the prevention of nutritional deficiencies. The National Academy of Sciences—National Research Council set up a Food and Nutrition Board to provide a list of Recommended Daily Dietary Allowances (RDA) for nutrients thought to be essential to meet the needs of the average person in good health living in the United States (Fig. 6-1). The amounts of nutrients are not sufficient for individuals with chronic illnesses or people under extreme stress. The allowances are reviewed periodically, the last time in 1968. These dietary allowances can be used in planning and prescribing adequate diets for persons. The dietronics nutritional evaluation is based upon this standard.

Other countries have RDA that differ from each other, depending upon the climates and the life styles of their population.

Minimum Daily Requirements

The Minimum Daily Requirement (MDR) is a dietary standard devised by the Food and Drug Administration. This standard appears on the packaging of food and is what the patient is familiar with, but he does not recognize its full significance. The MDR is the minimal amount of a nutrient of which less would produce deficiency symptoms such as scurvy (vitamin C deficiency) and pellagra (niacin deficiency). The MDR is an amount less than the recommended dietary allowance and should not be used as a guide for the adequate diet. On December 31, 1974, new U.S. Recommended Daily Allowances (U.S.R.D.A.) will go into effect. This set of standards has been established by the Food and Drug Administration and is derived from the values of nutrients (RDA) as set

FOOD AND NUTRITION BOARD, NATIONAL ACADEMY OF SCIENCES–NATIONAL RESEARCH COUNCIL
RECOMMENDED DAILY DIETARY ALLOWANCES,[a] REVISED 1968
Designed for the maintenance of good nutrition of practically all healthy people in the U.S.A.

	Age[b] (years) From / Up to	Weight (kg)	(lbs)	Height cm	(in.)	kcal	Protein (gm)	Vitamin A Activity (IU)	Vitamin D (IU)	Vitamin E Activity (IU)	Ascorbic Acid (mg)	Folacin (mg)	Niacin (mg equiv)[d]	Riboflavin (mg)	Thiamin (mg)	Vitamin B6 (mg)	Vitamin B12 (µg)	Calcium (g)	Phosphorus (g)	Iodine (µg)	Iron (mg)	Magnesium (mg)
Infants	0–1/6	4	9	55	22	kg × 120	kg × 2.2[f]	1,500	400	5	35	0.05	5	0.4	0.2	0.2	1.0	0.4	0.2	25	6	40
	1/6–1/2	7	15	63	25	kg × 110	kg × 2.0[f]	1,500	400	5	35	0.05	7	0.5	0.4	0.3	1.5	0.5	0.4	40	10	60
	1/2–1	9	20	72	28	kg × 100	kg × 1.8[f]	1,500	400	5	35	0.1	8	0.6	0.5	0.4	2.0	0.6	0.5	45	15	70
Children	1–2	12	26	81	32	1,100	25	2,000	400	10	40	0.1	8	0.6	0.6	0.5	2.0	0.7	0.7	55	15	100
	2–3	14	31	91	36	1,250	25	2,000	400	10	40	0.2	8	0.7	0.6	0.6	2.5	0.8	0.8	60	15	150
	3–4	16	35	100	39	1,400	30	2,500	400	10	40	0.2	9	0.8	0.7	0.7	3	0.8	0.8	70	10	200
	4–6	19	42	110	43	1,600	30	2,500	400	10	40	0.2	11	0.9	0.8	0.9	4	0.8	0.8	80	10	200
	6–8	23	51	121	48	2,000	35	3,500	400	15	40	0.2	13	1.1	1.0	1.0	4	0.9	0.9	100	10	250
	8–10	28	62	131	52	2,200	40	3,500	400	15	40	0.3	15	1.2	1.1	1.2	5	1.0	1.0	110	10	250
Males	10–12	35	77	140	55	2,500	45	4,500	400	20	40	0.4	17	1.3	1.3	1.4	5	1.2	1.2	125	10	300
	12–14	43	95	151	59	2,700	50	5,000	400	20	45	0.4	18	1.4	1.4	1.6	5	1.4	1.4	135	18	350
	14–18	59	130	170	67	3,000	60	5,000	400	25	55	0.4	20	1.5	1.5	1.8	5	1.4	1.4	150	18	400
	18–22	67	147	175	69	2,800	60	5,000	—	30	60	0.4	18	1.6	1.4	2.0	5	0.8	0.8	140	10	400
	22–35	70	154	175	69	2,800	65	5,000	—	30	60	0.4	18	1.7	1.4	2.0	5	0.8	0.8	140	10	350
	35–55	70	154	173	68	2,600	65	5,000	—	30	60	0.4	17	1.7	1.3	2.0	5	0.8	0.8	125	10	350
	55–75+	70	154	171	67	2,400	65	5,000	—	30	60	0.4	14	1.7	1.2	2.0	6	0.8	0.8	110	10	350
Females	10–12	35	77	142	56	2,250	50	4,500	400	20	40	0.4	15	1.3	1.1	1.4	5	1.2	1.2	110	18	300
	12–14	44	97	154	61	2,300	50	5,000	400	20	45	0.4	15	1.4	1.2	1.6	5	1.3	1.3	115	18	350
	14–16	52	114	157	62	2,400	55	5,000	400	25	50	0.4	16	1.4	1.2	1.8	5	1.3	1.3	120	18	350
	16–18	54	119	160	63	2,300	55	5,000	400	25	50	0.4	15	1.5	1.2	2.0	5	1.3	1.3	115	18	350
	18–22	58	128	163	64	2,000	55	5,000	400	25	55	0.4	13	1.5	1.0	2.0	5	0.8	0.8	100	18	350
	22–35	58	128	163	64	2,000	55	5,000	—	25	55	0.4	13	1.5	1.0	2.0	5	0.8	0.8	100	18	300
	35–55	58	128	160	63	1,850	55	5,000	—	25	55	0.4	13	1.5	1.0	2.0	5	0.8	0.8	90	18	300
	55–75+	58	128	157	62	1,700	55	5,000	—	25	55	0.4	13	1.5	1.0	2.0	6	0.8	0.8	80	18	300
Pregnancy						+200	65	6,000	400	30	60	0.8	15	1.8	+0.1	2.5	8	+0.4	+0.4	125	18	450
Lactation						+1,000	75	8,000	400	30	60	0.5	20	2.0	+0.5	2.5	6	+0.5	+0.5	150	18	450

[a] The allowance levels are intended to cover individual variations among most normal persons as they live in the United States under usual environmental stresses. The recommended allowances can be attained with a variety of common foods, providing other nutrients for which human requirements have been less well defined. See text for more-detailed discussion of allowances and of nutrients not tabulated.

Entries on lines for age range 22–35 years represent the reference man and woman at age 22. All other entries represent allowances for the midpoint of the specified age range.

[c] The folacin allowances refer to dietary sources as determined by *Lactobacillus casei* assay. Pure forms of folacin may be effective in doses less than 1/4 of the RDA.

[d] Niacin equivalents include dietary sources of the vitamin itself plus 1 mg equivalent for each 60 mg of dietary tryptophan.

[f] Assumes protein equivalent to human milk. For proteins not 100 percent utilized factors should be increased proportionately.

FIG. 6-1. Recommended Daily Dietary Allowances, Revised 1968 (courtesy of the National Research Council, Food and Nutrition Board).

forth by the National Research Council. These standards will be used to implement the provisions of the new regulations pertaining to nutritional labeling and dietary supplements and will replace the MDR.

Basic Four Food Groups

The Basic Four Food Groups scheme is used to select food and plan meals.

In 1958 the basic four food groups were adopted by the Department of Agriculture, replacing the basic seven food groups. It is a simple grouping of foods of similar nutrient value. The number of servings per day as suggested by this guide supplies approximately 1250 calories and 75 to 100 per cent of the recommended dietary allowances of the major nutrients except iron. The milk group provides approximately three fourths of the calcium, half the riboflavin, one fourth of the protein, one sixth of the vitamin A. Meat Group: two fifths to half of the protein, three to four fifths of the niacin, one sixth to one third of the iron, one fourth

of the thiamine and riboflavin, half the vitamin A. Fruits and vegetable group: all the vitamin C, three fourths of the vitamin A, one sixth to one fourth of the iron and thiamine. Bread-cereal group, enriched or whole grain: one fourth of the thiamine, one sixth to one fourth of the iron, and over one third of the niacin.

The foods listed in the four food groups used in the recommended servings are considered foundation foods. Additional servings and additional foods may be added to meet the nutritive as well as the caloric needs of the individual. A Guide to Good Eating (Fig. 6-2) is simple and easy to apply in everyday living.

Milk Group. Whole milk and fortified milk provide vitamins A and D. Vitamin D–fortified milk is the chief source of vitamin D in the diet. Nonfat milks should be fortified with vitamins A and D as these nutrients are lacking because of the removal of butter fats. Evaporated milk is whole milk in which about half the water has been removed.

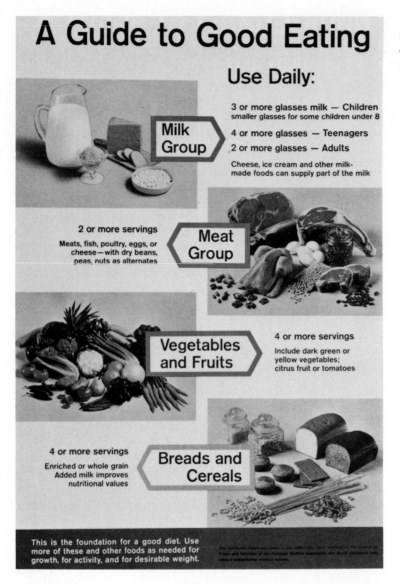

A Guide to Good Eating

Use Daily:

Milk Group

3 or more glasses milk — Children
smaller glasses for some children under 8

4 or more glasses — Teenagers

2 or more glasses — Adults

Cheese, ice cream and other milk-
made foods can supply part of the milk

Meat Group

2 or more servings

Meats, fish, poultry, eggs, or
cheese—with dry beans,
peas, nuts as alternates

Vegetables and Fruits

4 or more servings

Include dark green or
yellow vegetables;
citrus fruit or tomatoes

Breads and Cereals

4 or more servings

Enriched or whole grain
Added milk improves
nutritional values

This is the foundation for a good diet. Use
more of these and other foods as needed for
growth, for activity, and for desirable weight.

Fig. 6-2. A Guide to Good Eating (courtesy of the National Dairy Council).

It is rich in calcium and protein. Condensed milk is milk in which approximately 42 per cent sugar has been added before the evaporating process.

Cultured buttermilk is made from skim milk. Yogurt is made from concentrated whole milk fermented with a mixture of one or more strains of such organisms as *Streptococcus thermophilus.* Acidophilus milk is made of skim milk cultured with *Lactobacillus acidophilus.*

Cheese is made from the curd of milk and is high in calcium, protein, and riboflavin. Cheddar cheese is made of whole milk. Processed cheese is a blend of various cheeses plus an emulsifier and is pasteurized. Cottage cheese is made from pasteurized skim milk and is of high quality protein. Cream cheese is made of whole milk with cream added and is high in fat and vitamin A.

Milk and milk products are the main source of calcium. They particularly supply protein, vitamin A, and vitamin B$_2$ (ribo-flavin). Common servings of foods and their milk equivalents in calcium are:

1 inch cube cheddar cheese = the amount of calcium in ½ cup of milk

½ cup cottage cheese = the amount of calcium in ⅓ cup of milk

2 tablespoons cream cheese = the amount of calcium in 1 tablespoon milk

½ cup ice cream = the amount of calcium in ¼ cup milk

The number of servings recommended per day in terms of whole fluid milk:

Children under 9 years, 2 to 3 cups

Children 9 to 12 years, 3 or more cups

Teenagers, 4 or more cups

Adults, 2 or more cups

Pregnant women, 3 or more cups

Nursing mothers, 4 or more cups

Meat Group. Lamb, beef, veal, pork, organ meats, poultry, eggs, fish and shell-fish, dried beans, dried peas, nuts, peanuts, and peanut butter. These foods contain pro-tein, iron, niacin, thiamine, riboflavin, and vitamin A. Eggs and meat, especially liver, are important for iron and the B vitamins. Pork is important for the B vitamins, espe-cially thiamine. The legumes, dried beans and dried peas, and nuts are good sources of iron and thiamine but should be supple-mented with animal protein to make the vegetable protein more useful to the body.

The following foods represent a serving equal to 2 to 3 ounces of lean cooked meat, poultry, or fish without bone:

2 eggs

1 cup cooked lentils

1 cup cooked dry beans

4 tablespoons peanut butter

Two servings per day are recommended from the meat group, and they should be served several times throughout the day. Suggested food selection:

1 egg daily or at least 3 to 5 per week

Liver, heart, kidney, or sweetbreads once a week

Other kinds of meat, fish, poultry, or cheese four to five or more times a week

Dried beans, dried peas, nuts, or peanut butter served with milk or cheese

Fruit and *Vegetable Group.* These foods primarily provide vitamin C and vitamin A as well as trace amounts of other nutrients.

Good sources of vitamin C and the amount considered a serving are:

½ grapefruit, ¾ cup grapefruit juice

1 medium orange, ¾ cup orange juice

½ large cantaloupe

1 cup strawberries

¾ cup broccoli

1½ cups cabbage, raw, shredded.

Fair sources of vitamin C are honeydew melon, lemon, tangerine, watermelon, asparagus tips, collards, garden cress, kale, mustard greens, medium potato and sweet potato cooked in the jacket, spinach, toma-toes, and turnip greens.

Sources of vitamin A are the dark green and deep yellow vegetables and a few fruits —the deeper the green or yellow, the higher the source of vitamin A: Broccoli, chard, collards, cress, kale, spinach, turnip greens, all dark green leaves. Apricots, cantaloupe, carrots, mango, persimmon, pumpkin, sweet potato, and winter squash.

The green leafy vegetables also supply vitamins E and K, calcium, and iron. The size of a serving is ½ cup or a portion that is ordinarily served such as 1 medium apple, 1 banana. Four or more servings are recom-mended daily, one of which is a good source of vitamin C. Dark green or deep yellow vegetables or yellow fruits are recommended three or four times a week.

Bread and Cereal Group. This group in-cludes breads, cooked cereals, ready-to-eat cereals, cornmeal, crackers, flour, grits, macaroni, spaghetti, noodles, rice, rolled oats, quick breads and baked goods if made from grains or enriched flour, and parboiled rice and wheat. These foods supply iron, thiamine, riboflavin, and protein, but the quality and quantity are less than in foods of the milk and meat groups.

The whole-grain cereals and breads supply the necessary nutrients, whereas the refined

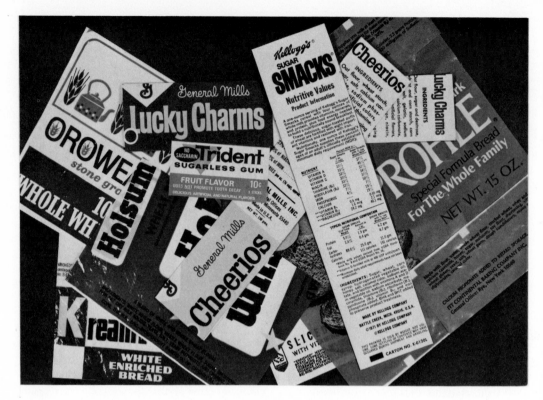

FIG. 6-3. A display of labels.

breads and cereals are lower in nutrients. The size of servings:

  1 slice bread
  1 ounce ready-to-eat cereal
  ½ to ¾ cup cooked cereal, cornmeal, grits, macaroni, rice, or spaghetti

If cereal is chosen, the recommended number of servings is four daily. Five servings daily are recommended if cereal is not used.

Economic factors play a major role in the foods that are eaten. Many times the cheaper foods are used in greater abundance without thought being given to their nutritive value. This tends to result in clinical and subclinical deficiencies. Considering the milk group; the nonfat milk solids cost less than fresh milk. They should be fortified with vitamin A and vitamin D. Evaporated milk is another economical form of milk.

The foods in the meat group are the most expensive. However, the less expensive grades and cuts of meats have the same nutritive value as the more expensive cuts. The organ meats have high nutritional value. The dried peas and beans, which are incomplete protein, are economical foods and when prepared with small amounts of meat or dairy products complete the protein to assist in meeting the amino acid requirement of the body. Such dishes are pea soup with ham and chili con carne. For the protein to be used most effectively in the body, it should be divided into small portions and served at the various meals throughout the day, for example, two eggs at breakfast; a tuna fish sandwich at lunch; beef stew at dinner.

The foods in the fruit and vegetable groups can be fresh, canned, or frozen. The fresh foods can be expensive in the northern states where the growing season is short. The distance they must travel increases the cost. The nutritive value of produce can also be

FIG. 6-4. Scoreboard from pamphlet *How Do You Score on Nutrition?* (courtesy of the Vitamin Information Bureau).

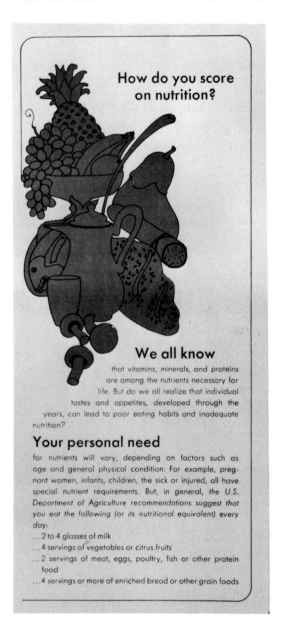

How do you score on nutrition?

We all know

that vitamins, minerals, and proteins are among the nutrients necessary for life. But do we all realize that individual tastes and appetites, developed through the years, can lead to poor eating habits and inadequate nutrition?

Your personal need

for nutrients will vary, depending on factors such as age and general physical condition. For example, pregnant women, infants, children, the sick or injured, all have special nutrient requirements. But, in general, *the U.S. Department of Agriculture recommendations suggest that you eat the following (or its nutritional equivalent) every day:*

...2 to 4 glasses of milk

...4 servings of vegetables or citrus fruits

...2 servings of meat, eggs, poultry, fish or other protein food

...4 servings or more of enriched bread or other grain foods

decreased because of the time between harvest and serving at the table.

The foods in the bread and cereal group are the most economical and must be selected with the greatest care. The highly processed and refined foods can be high in calories and low in nutritive value. The labels of these foods must be read carefully.

Some nationalities and ethnic groups have specific food patterns that affect their selection of food. The Orientals use rice. In the northern United States, wheat flour, bread, spinach, kale, and winter squash are in common use. In the southern states cornmeal, grits, rice, collards, mustard greens, turnip greens, and dried peas are used more. The Latin Americans use cornmeal. The Italians use spaghetti, macaroni, and other pastas.

MISCELLANEOUS AIDS IN
PLANNING AN ADEQUATE DIET
Food Labels

Food labels provide a visual aid that can be used to discuss the minimum daily requirement as compared to the recommended dietary allowance. Two boxes of dry cereal can be compared, one cereal being sugar coated, to which 100 per cent of the MDR of certain nutrients has been added, and the other an unsugared cereal with lesser amounts of nutrients.

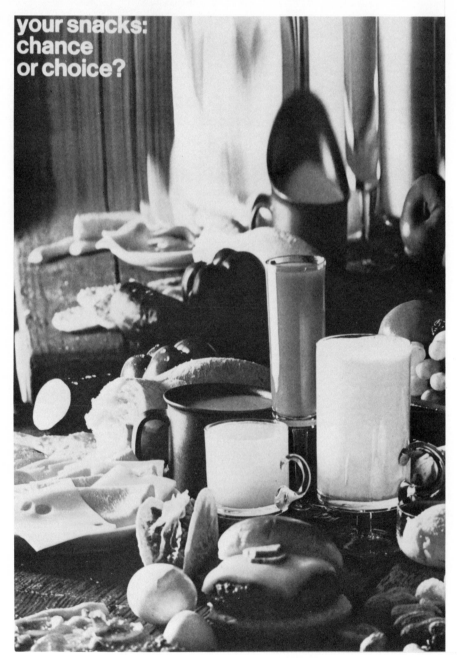

FIG. 6-5. Your Snacks: Chance or Choice? (courtesy of the National Dairy Council).

HIDDEN SUGAR: CARBOHYDRATE EVALUATION

The approximate refined carbohydrate content of popular foods in amounts equivalent to teaspoonsful of sugar was compiled from current publications on food values:

Candy runs from 75% to 85% sugar. Popular candy bars are likely to weigh 1 to 5 oz. and may contain 5 to 20 teaspoons sugar.

....

t = teaspoon

Chocolate creams	35 to 1 lb.	2	t sugar
Chocolate fudge	1½" sq. 15 to 1 lb.	4	t sugar
Butterscotch	1" x 1"	1	t sugar
Chocolate mints	1 medium (20 to 1 lb.)	3	t sugar
Life Savers	1 usual size	1/3	t sugar
Chewing gum	1 stick	½	t sugar

....

Chocolate cake	2-layer icing (1/12 cake)	15	t sugar
Angel Food	1 piece (1/12 of large cake)	6	t sugar
Cream puff - iced	1 average custard filled	5	t sugar
Doughnut, plain	3" diameter	4	t sugar
Macaroons	1 large or 2 small	3	t sugar
Gingersnaps	1 medium	1	t sugar
Molasses cookies	3½" diameter	2	t sugar
Brownies	2" x 2" x 3/4"	3	t sugar

....

Custard	½ cup	4	t sugar
Gelatin	½ cup	4	t sugar

....

Icecream	1/8 quart	2 to 3	t sugar
Sherbet	1/8 quart	4 to 6	t sugar

....

Apple pie	1/6 medium pie	12	t sugar
Cherry pie	1/6 medium pie	14	t sugar
Raisin pie	1/6 medium pie	13	t sugar
Pumpkin pie	1/6 medium pie	10	t sugar

CARBOHYDRATE EVALUATION

....

T = Tablespoon   t = teaspoon

Jam	1 T level or 1 heaping t	3	t sugar
Jelly	1 T level or 1 heaping t	2½	t sugar
Syrup, maple	1 T level	2½	t sugar
Honey	1 T level	3	t sugar

....

Chocolate, all milk	1 cup, 5 oz. milk	6	t sugar
Cocoa, all milk	1 cup, 5 oz. milk	4	t sugar
Egg nog, all milk	1 glass, 8 oz. milk	4½	t sugar

....

Soft Drinks	1 bottle, 6 oz.	4 and 1/3	t sugar
Gingerale	6 oz. glass	3 and 1/3	t sugar
Sweet cider	6 oz. glass	4 ½	t sugar

....

Fruit cocktail	½ cup	5	t sugar
Orange juice	½ cup	2	t sugar
Pineapple juice (unsweetened)	½ cup	2½	t sugar
Grapefruit juice (unsweetened)	½ cup	2	t sugar
Grape juice (commercial)	½ cup	3 and 2/3	t sugar

....

Peaches, canned in syrup	2 halves, 1 T juice	3½	t sugar
Apple sauce (no sugar)	½ cup	2	t sugar
Rhubarb, stewed	½ cup sweetened	8	t sugar

....

Apricots, dried	4 to 6 halves	4	t sugar
Prunes, dried	3 to 4 medium	4	t sugar
Dates, dried	3 to 4 pitted	4½	t sugar
Figs, dried	1½ to 2 small	4	t sugar
Raisins	½ cup	4	t sugar

****

FIG. 6-6. Hidden Sugar: Carbohydrate Evaluation (courtesy of the Dental Health Unit, Department of Social and Health Services, the State of Washington).

Ingredients can also be analyzed and discussed. Food companies usually list the ingredients in order of proportion, the largest being first.

It is suggested that the patient be selective in purchasing. He should read labels (Fig. 6-3). Only breads and cereals that contain 100 per cent whole wheat or that have been enriched or restored should be used. This includes rolls, buns, cereals, crackers, pancake flour, bakery-made pastries of all varieties, macaroni, spaghetti and rice.

Pamphlets, Pictures and Filmstrips

Your Food: Chance or Choice? is a pamphlet written for the teenager. It discusses food selection in relation to common eating habits.

A Boy and His Physique and *A Girl and Her Figure* are booklets written for the teenager that tell about growth patterns, eating habits, and food selection in relationship to individual needs. This information provides insight into youth development, exercise, and body requirements and is of interest to parents as well as the teenager.

How Do You Score on Nutrition? (Fig. 6-4) is a pamphlet containing a day-by-day check list of the intake of essential nutrients. Its use by the patient indicates to him the specific nutrients lacking if certain foods are omitted from the diet.

Your Snacks: Chance or Choice? (Fig 6-5) is an excellent picture in color of foods suitable for between-meal eating. An attractive picture of food is a more persuasive means of convincing the patient to alter his food selection than discussion alone.

Hidden Sugar: Carbohydrate Evaluation (Fig. 6-6) allows the patient to see and understand where sugar can enter into the diet. The amount of sugar in foods can be further emphasized by placing sugar in test tubes that represent the approximate content of refined carbohydrate in various popular foods such as a candy bar, Life Saver, carbonated beverage, and chocolate milk (Fig. 6-7).

Judy's Family Food Notebook, a filmstrip, presents the subject of nutrition to the

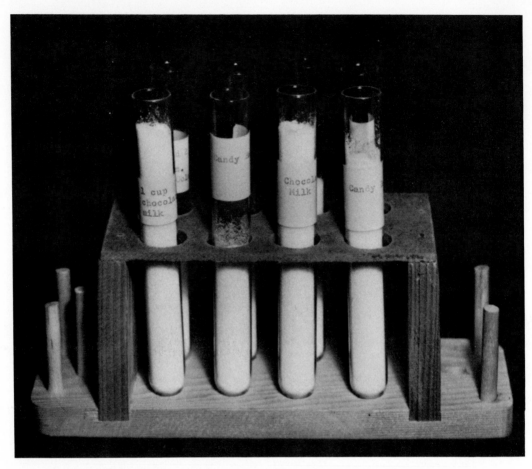

FIG. 6-7. Test tubes filled with sugar representing the carbohydrate content of popular foods.

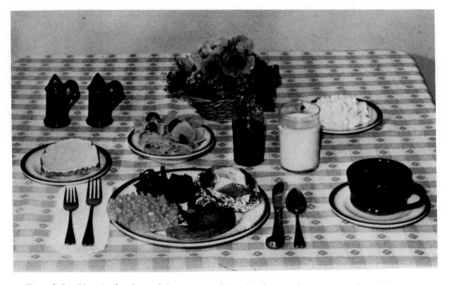

FIG. 6-8. Plastic food models arranged in the form of a prepared meal (courtesy of NASCO).

young patient. It is approximately 15 minutes in length and is in cartoon form and programmed for children approximately 5 through 12 years of age. The story is of a child who makes a notebook about the foods in the basic four food groups. It is without sound, a booklet comes with the filmstrip, and the story must be taped. The advantage of this is that the message can be reworded to fit the needs of the preventive practice.

Vitamins and You is a filmstrip shown to the junior and senior high school students. It tells the history of vitamins, their discovery, and how they function in the body. The patient advances the filmstrip by using a pushbutton from the projector as he hears the cue. This is a real treat for the young patient. Children as young as 5 or 6 years will complete the filmstrip properly.

Food Models

Plastic food models, are used by children from age 5 to 17 to arrange a proper breakfast, lunch, and dinner (Fig. 6-8). The children count the number of servings per food group in the three meals they have planned. As the food is arranged and rearranged by the child, the balanced diet is discussed. This becomes a meaningful visual learning experience.

Some parents have continued these experiences at home by playing games with their children during meals by counting the number of servings eaten. This will motivate the child to eat perhaps one more serving of vegetable or another portion of meat.

Aids Used to Meet the Needs of the Patient

The 5-Day Food Diary. This diary (Fig. 6-9) is used to identify the refined carbo-

	Date	Amount	Date	Amount
	Before Breakfast		Before Breakfast	
	Breakfast		Breakfast	
	Between Meals		Between Meals	
	Lunch		Lunch	
FOOD DIARY				
	Between Meals		Between Meals	
	Dinner		Dinner	
Dr. A. G. Dingerson 513 N. Morrison Rd. Vancouver, Washington 98664 Telephone 694-5211				
	After Dinner		After Dinner	

FIG. 6-9. Food Diary (adapted from earlier suggestions by The University of Texas Dental Branch at Houston).

PLEASE PRINT CLEARLY

PATIENT'S NAME			DATE	
	FIRST	LAST		

ADDRESS						
	NO.	STREET	CITY	STATE		ZIP
AGE	SEX	PREGNANT? LACTATING?	HT	WT		

——————————— DO NOT WRITE IN THIS SPACE ———————————

TO THE PATIENT:

Read all instructions before answering questions. Complete PARTS A, B, and C. Include all eating between meals as well as regular meals when answering questions. Recheck your answers. The accuracy of this evaluation depends on the accuracy of your answers.

part a: READ EACH QUESTION CAREFULLY AND ANSWER BY CHECKING THE APPROPRIATE BOX OR FILLING IN THE BLANK.

1) Do you generally eat portions that are: ☐ large ☐ average ☐ small

2) Do you often eat seconds? ☐ yes ☐ no

3) How do you like steak? ☐ rare ☐ medium ☐ well done

4) Do you avoid or cut fat from your meat? ☐ yes ☐ no

5) Do you prefer your bacon to be very crisp? ☐ yes ☐ no

6) Do you like gravies on meat and/or sauces on vegetables? ☐ yes ☐ no

7) Are your margarine and oils: ☐ polyunsaturated ☐ pay no attention

8) How many packs of cigarettes do you smoke daily? _____

9) What kind of bread do you eat? ☐ whole grain ☐ white ☐ both

10) Do you add salt to your food at the table? ☐ yes ☐ no

11) Do you use iodized salt? ☐ yes ☐ no

12) What kind of fruit do you eat? ☐ fresh ☐ canned ☐ sugar free

13) Do you prefer doughnuts: ☐ plain ☐ iced or filled ☐ do not eat

14) How many bottles of soft drinks do you drink daily? _____

15) Are these soft drinks: ☐ sugar free ☐ low calorie ☐ regular

16) Do you eat sugar-coated cereal? ☐ yes ☐ no

17) How many teaspoons sugar do you use on your cereal? _____

18) Do you prefer pancakes with: ☐ syrup or jam ☐ honey ☐ do not eat

19) How many cups of coffee, tea, or a substitute do you drink daily? _____

20) How many teaspoons of sugar do you use in your coffee or tea? _____

21) Do you drink your coffee or tea with: ☐ cream or half and half ☐ milk ☐ imitation cream ☐ black

22) If you eat between meals is it usually during: ☐ morning ☐ afternoon ☐ night ☐ do not snack

23) Are your snacks most often: ☐ potato chips, corn curls, etc. ☐ fruit or vegetables ☐ cheese and crackers ☐ sandwich ☐ cookies, sweets ☐ do not snack

*24) Do you use food supplements? ☐ yes ☐ no

Do you get them from: ☐ your doctor ☐ drug or grocery store ☐ health food store

Which supplements do you use? ☐ Multiple ☐ B Complex ☐ Iron ☐ Calcium ☐ Vitamin A ☐ Vitamin C ☐ Vitamin E

*Values of nutrients supplied by food supplements are not included in this evaluation except on research projects where provision has been made in advance.

%RDA is the percentage of the nutrient in the diet of the Recommended Dietary Allowance for the designated age and sex of the patient. RDA's established by the National Research Council (1968), or if not established the consensus of medical literature is used. If age is not indicated, 22–34 years is assumed. If sex is not indicated, male is assumed.

Deviations from the recommended dietary allowances are significant only in terms of the patient's total health status as determined by the physician and should not be the ONLY measure of nutritional adequacy. USE CARE IN INTERPRETING THESE FIGURES, for your dentist or physician may determine needs greater or less for individuals.

PROTEIN allowance is estimated on a basis of protein intake that is 70% of ideal quality and should be increased for poor quality of protein foods and amino acid pattern. VITAMIN E requirements increase with amount of polyunsaturated fats. VITAMIN B6 requirements may increase with increased protein intake. VITAMIN B1 and NIACIN requirements increase with increased caloric intake.

FIG. 6-10. Nutritional evaluation questionnaire (courtesy of Dietronics).

part b:

● HOW OFTEN DO YOU EAT THE FOLLOWING FOODS? PUT A CHECK MARK IN THE COLUMN <u>CLOSEST</u> TO YOUR EATING HABITS. <u>DO NOT</u> PUT A CHECK OR COMMENT IF EATEN LESS THAN TWICE MONTHLY.

● <u>IF YOU EAT DIFFERENT PORTIONS THAN WHAT ARE LISTED</u>, WRITE IN YOUR PORTION IN THE SPACE PROVIDED AND CHECK THE COLUMN CLOSEST TO HOW OFTEN YOU EAT THE PORTION YOU SPECIFY.

● BE SURE TO INCLUDE SNACKS WHEN ANSWERING THIS PART.

FOOD	AMT PER SERVING		OFFICE USE	3 TIMES DAILY	TWICE DAILY	ONCE DAILY	3 TIMES WEEKLY	ONCE WEEKLY	TWICE MONTHLY
CEREAL (1 CUP)		1							
OATMEAL (1 CUP)		2							
BREAD (2 SLICES)		3							
PANCAKES (2)		4							
CAKE (1 PC.), COOKIES (3)		5							
PUMPKIN PIE (1/6 PIE)		6							
OTHER PIE (1/6 PIE)		7							
ROLLS, BUNS, MUFFINS (2)		8							
CRACKERS, ANY KIND (4)		9							
MACARONI AND CHEESE (1 CUP)		10							
SPAGHETTI (1 CUP)		11							
SWEET ROLL (1), DOUGHNUTS (2)		12							
RICE (1 CUP COOKED)		13							
BEEF OR LAMB, ANY FORM (5 oz)		14							
BEEF STEW (1 CUP)		15							
HAM, PORK (4 oz)		16							
CHILI, LUNCHEON MEATS (3 oz)		17							
LIVERWURST SAUSAGE (2 oz)		18							
LIVER (BEEF OR CHICKEN) (2 oz)		19							
KIDNEY, SWEETBREADS, HEART (3 oz)		20							
BACON (2 STRIPS)		21							
SHRIMP, OYSTERS, CRAB, CLAMS, LOBSTER (3/4 CUP)		22							
FISH, INCLUDING TUNA FISH (4 oz)		23							
CHICKEN, TURKEY, FOWL (5 oz)		24							
EGGS (2)		25							
SARDINES (1/2 CAN)		26							
ANY CREAMED SOUPS (1/2 CUP)		27							
WHOLE MILK (1 CUP)		28							
BUTTERMILK OR SKIMMED (1 CUP)		29							
CHEESE, EXCEPT COTTAGE (1 oz) (INCL. BLUE CHEESE DRESSINGS)		30							

FOOD	AMT PER SERVING		OFFICE USE	3 TIMES DAILY	TWICE DAILY	ONCE DAILY	3 TIMES WEEKLY	ONCE WEEKLY	TWICE MONTHLY
COTTAGE CHEESE (1/2 CUP)		31							
ICE CREAM (1/3 CUP)		32							
BERRIES (EXCEPT FRESH STRAWBERRIES) (1 CUP)		33							
CITRUS (JUICE OR FRUIT), FRESH STRAWBERRIES (1 CUP)		34							
CANTALOUPE (1/2)		35							
OTHER FRUIT (1 PC. OR 1 CUP)		36							
TOMATO (RAW, CANNED) (1 CUP)		37							
VEGETABLE SOUP (1 CUP)		38							
SALAD (LETTUCE), COLE SLAW (1 CUP)		39							
GREEN PEPPER (1), BRUSSEL SPROUTS (1 CUP)		40							
SWEET POTATOES, YAMS (1)		41							
WHITE POTATOES (1)		42							
BEETS, ONIONS, RADISHES (1/2 CUP)		43							
BEANS, EXCEPT GREEN (3/4 CUP) (INCL. LENTILS, BAKED, ETC.)		44							
CAULIFLOWER (1 CUP)		45							
SUMMER SQUASH, ZUCCHINI (1 CUP)		46							
GREEN BEANS, CORN, PEAS (INCLUDE PEA SOUP) (1 CUP)		47							
CARROTS (1/2 CUP)		48							
SPINACH, CHARD (3/4 CUP)		49							
WINTER SQUASH, BEET GREENS (1 CUP)		50							
MUSTARD OR TURNIP GREENS, KALE (1 CUP)		51							
BROCCOLI (1 CUP)		52							
CANDY OTHER THAN CHOCOLATE (5 PC. HARD CANDY)		53							
CANDY BAR, CHOCOLATE (1)		54							
BUTTER (1 TBSP.)		55							
NUTS AND SEEDS (1/2 CUP), PEANUT BUTTER (1 TBSP.)		56							
MARGARINE (1 TBSP.)		57							
OIL DRESSINGS (FR. & ITAL.) (1 TBSP.)		58							
MAYONNAISE, 1000 ISLAND (1 TBSP.)		59							
ANY FRIED FOOD		60							

part c:

ENTER BELOW ANY OTHER FOODS REGULARLY EATEN WHICH HAVE NOT BEEN INCLUDED IN PART B. WRITE IN THE PORTION AND CHECK THE COLUMN CLOSEST TO YOUR EATING HABITS. BE SURE TO INCLUDE ALCOHOLIC BEVERAGES (SPECIFY WHAT KIND).

FOOD	AMT PER SERVING	OFFICE USE	3 TIMES DAILY	TWICE DAILY	ONCE DAILY	3 TIMES WEEKLY	ONCE WEEKLY	TWICE MONTHLY

FOOD	AMT PER SERVING	OFFICE USE	3 TIMES DAILY	TWICE DAILY	ONCE DAILY	3 TIMES WEEKLY	ONCE WEEKLY	TWICE MONTHLY

FIG. 6-11. Nutritional evaluation questionnaire (courtesy of Dietronics).

```
DENTAL PROFILE FOR:
                                ACTUAL       RECOMMENDED
                       %RDA     AMOUNT         (RDA)
GROSS NUTRIENTS
   PROTEIN             164       90.    GM     55.00
   CALORIES            131      2600.          2000.00
   CARBOHYDRATE                  330.   GM
   SUGAR                         36.    TSPS   KEEP LOW
VITAMINS
   A                   159      8000.   USPU   5000.00
   E                    71       18.    I.U.    25.00
   B-1                 117        1.2   MG       1.00
   B-2                 155        2.3   MG       1.50
   NIACIN              136       18.    MG      13.00
   B-6                 103        2.1   MG       2.00
   PANTOTHENIC ACID     72        7.3   MG      10.00
   B-12                166        8.3   MCGM     5.00
   C                   109       60.    MG      55.00
MINERALS
   CALCIUM             115      930.    MG     800.00
   MAGNESIUM            90      270.    MG     300.00
   PHOSPHORUS          160     1300.    MG     800.00
   IRON                 91       16.    MG      18.00
RATIOS
   RCAL/CAL*                     49%           KEEP LOW
   CALC/PHOS                      0.72
   *EQUIVALENT TO CALORIES FROM  64 TSPS SUGAR PER DAY

FOOD GROUPS - AVERAGE DAILY SERVINGS
                             ACTUAL     RECOMMENDED
   CEREAL                     4.6           4
   PROTEIN                    2.0           2
   VEG-FRUIT                  2.0           4
   DAIRY                      1.9           2

AVERAGE DAILY FOOD EXPOSURES
   PLAQUE FORMING             3.1         KEEP LOW
   FIRM NONPLAQUE FORMING     2.3         KEEP HIGH




COMMENT:

NUTRIENTS BELOW RDA

VITAMIN E
B-COMPLEX
```

FIG. 6-12. Nutritional evaluation printout (courtesy of Dietronics).

hydrates, specifically the sugar and flour foods. These foods feed the bacteria that produce decay. This diary is also used to separate the nutritious foods from the nonnutritious foods. If a nutritional evaluation such as Dietronics is not included in the program, the food diary can be used to determine the adequacy of the diet. From this history the patient identifies the foods he eats within the basic four food groups. He is able to analyze his eating pattern and food selection as well as plan meals that are more conducive to good health.

The written instructions on the form should be few and simple; otherwise, the patient will not read them. The days covered should include a Saturday, Sunday, or a holiday because the food choices and eating patterns vary on these days. Everything the patient eats and drinks and its approximate amount are recorded. If the adequacy of the diet is to be determined by this record, the size of servings becomes critical and should be handled accordingly.

Initially, the control therapist assists the patient in the recall of the foods he has eaten during the past 24 hours. No comment should be made concerning his selection of foods.

It is to be noted that there is no typical week. Many reasons will be given for this. Some women, rather than write down all the

FOODS HIGH IN ESSENTIAL NUTRIENTS

Foods listed in approximate amounts supplied by average servings, highest first and decreasing as reading down (Recommended daily allowances on rear – consult physician or dentist for details)

dietronics®

Box 35 Northridge California 91324
Phone (213) 882-7266

PROTEIN
Eggs
Milk, cheese
Fish
Chicken
Beef
Pork
Soybeans
Beans, peas
Nuts

FATS
Margarine
Butter
Peanut butter
Salad oils
Cream, cheese
Bacon, pork
Beef
Fish

CALCIUM
Cheese
Milk
Bread
Nuts
Legumes
Green leafy vegetables

IRON
Liver
Organ meats
Eggs
Legumes
Green leafy vegetables
Oysters

POTASSIUM
Green leafy vegetables
Legumes
Nuts
Cocoa
Vegetable juices

VITAMIN A
Carrots
Green leafy vegetables
Butter
Whole milk
Liver
Fish

VITAMIN B-1
Liver
Pork
Yeast
Organ meats
Whole grains
Bread
Wheat germ
Peanuts

VITAMIN B-2
Eggs
Liver
Yeast
Milk
Whole grains
Bread
Wheat germ

NIACIN
Yeast
Liver
Wheat bran
Peanuts
Beans

VITAMIN C
Citrus
Fresh fruits
Berries
Broccoli
Tomatoes
Green leafy vegetables
Baked potatoes
Turnips

VITAMIN B-6
Wheat germ
Kidney
Liver
Ham
Organ meats
Legumes
Peanuts

PANTOTHENIC ACID
Liver
Organ meats
Eggs
Yeast
Wheat bran
Legumes
Cereals

IODINE
Iodized salt
Shellfish
Ocean fish
Bacon

VITAMIN E
Margarine
Oil salad dressing
Vegetable oils
Eggs
Cereal germ

VITAMIN B-12
Liver
Organ meats
Oysters
Salmon
Eggs
Beef

TRYPTOPHANE
Soy milk
Fish
Beef
Soy flour
Organ meats
Shellfish
Eggs

PHENYLALANINE
Beef
Fish
Eggs
Whole wheat
Shellfish
Organ meats
Soya
Milk

LEUCINE
Beef
Fish
Organ meats
Eggs
Soya
Shellfish
Whole wheat
Milk
Liver

ISO-LEUCINE
Fish
Beef
Organ meats
Eggs
Shellfish
Whole wheat
Soya
Milk

LYSINE
Fish
Beef
Organ meats
Shellfish
Eggs
Soya
Milk
Liver

VALINE
Beef
Fish
Organ meats
Eggs
Soya
Milk
Whole wheat
Liver

METHIONINE
Fish
Beef
Shellfish
Eggs
Milk
Liver
Whole wheat
Cheese

THREONINE
Fish
Beef
Organ meats
Eggs
Shellfish
Soya
Liver

POLYUNSAT. FATTY ACIDS
Margarine from safflower, corn, soy (non hydrogenated)
Corn oil (35%)
Safflower oil (70%)
Peanut oil (28%)
Soybean oil (50%)
Cottonseed oil (50%)
Lard (10%)

MAGNESIUM
Soya flour
Whole wheat
Oatmeal
Peas
Brown rice
Whole corn
Beans
Nuts

PHOSPHORUS
Highest dietary sources include protein foods such as
Soya flour
Whole wheat
Oatmeal
Peas
Brown rice
Whole corn
Beans
Nuts

SODIUM
The greatest portion of sodium is provided by table salt and salt used in cooking. Foods high in sodium include:
Dried beef
Ham
Canned corned beef
Bacon
Wheat breads
Salted crackers
Flaked breakfast cereals
Olives
Cheese
Butter
Margarine
Sausage
Dried fish
Canned vegetables
Shellfish and salt water fish
Raw celery

Refs: – Wohl & Goodhart, Modern Nutrition in Health & Disease, Lea & Febiger 1964; – Heinz Handbook of Nutrition; – Bicknell & Prescott, The Vitamins in Medicine, 3rd Ed. Heinemann, 1953; – U. S. Dept. Agriculture Food Tables; – Bowes & Church, Food Values, J. B. Lippincott 10th Ed.; – Kleiner & Orten, Biochemistry, 7th Ed. C. V. Mosby Co., 1966.

FORM D2109

FIG. 6-13. Foods high in essential nutrients (courtesy of Dietronics).

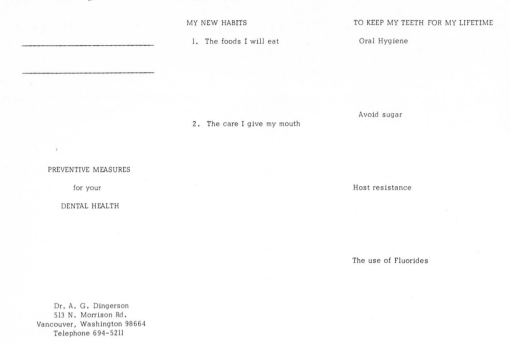

MY NEW HABITS

1. The foods I will eat

_____

_____

2. The care I give my mouth

PREVENTIVE MEASURES

for your

DENTAL HEALTH

TO KEEP MY TEETH FOR MY LIFETIME

Oral Hygiene

Avoid sugar

Host resistance

The use of Fluorides

Dr. A. G. Dingerson
513 N. Morrison Rd.
Vancouver, Washington 98664
Telephone 694-5211

FIG. 6-14. Preventive Measures for your Dental Health, a personal worksheet (adapted from earlier suggestions by The University of Texas Dental Branch at Houston).

"junk" they are eating, will decide to go on a diet. People will do three things to "shape up": have a physical exam, have a dental checkup, and go on a diet. If they choose to go on a diet at this time, the diary will in all probability not correlate with the patient's size or his oral conditions. However, this may be the stimulation necessary to improve food selections. The opportunity must be seized and adjustments made so the patient will understand the foods that relate to the mechanism of disease.

The Clinical Nutritional Evaluation — Dietronics.[1] The patient completes the information in a special questionnaire (Fig. 6-10, 6-11) concerning the frequency of the foods he eats. The information is interpreted through data processing. The results are tabulated and compared to the Recommended Dietary Allowances set up by the Food and Nutrition Board of the National Academy of Sciences.

The types of evaluations available to the dentist are Total Diet, Dental Profile, Meta-

bolic Profile and Medical Profile. The Dental Profile is used in the control program in this text.

The patient's resistance plays a role in periodontal disease. This resistance is lowered and becomes a susceptibility factor if essential vitamins and minerals are absent from the diet. The purpose of the Dietronics service is to make the patient realize the need for and the significance of nutrients to sustain health and make him feel good. He must respect the foods he eats and the reasons for eating them if he is going to be motivated to improve his food habits. Patients are very receptive and appreciative of this service. It is highly motivational.

The nutrients and related information are listed on the left of the computer printout that is returned from data processing (Fig. 6-12). Reading from left to right, the first column of figures indicates the percentage of the recommended dietary allowance for each nutrient. The second column of figures gives an estimated daily amount expressed in milligrams, grams, or units of nutrients in the diet, as determined by the foods that

[1] This is a service provided by a division of Hanson Research Corporation, Northridge, Calif. 91324.

MY DENTAL CONCERN

Decay
Gum Disease

WHY!

_____

Food   +   Bacteria _make_ Acid
Sugar
Starch

Acid   +   Tooth _lead_ Decay

Irritants + Gums ---- Gum Disease
                  to

_____

Forms of sugar

Liquid
Solid
Sticky, retentive

_____

SUGAR EATEN BETWEEN MEALS
         CAUSES DECAY

_____

Best time to eat sugar is during and
at the end of meals

_____

30 seconds after eating sugar, acid
is formed. Sugar remains in my
mouth _____ minutes

If bacterial plaque is organized,
decay may take place

Modified Snyder Test results _____

FOOD PATTERN

Number of meals I eat a day _____

Number of snacks I eat a day _____

My favorite snacks _____

The main decay producing foods shown
in my Five Day Food Diary _____

The number of times my teeth were
exposed to decay producing foods
during this five day period _____

The number of times my teeth were
exposed to decay producing foods
between meals during this five day
period   _____

                          _____

The number of times my teeth were
exposed to decay producing foods
during and at the end of meals
during this five day period _____

                          _____

Snack food is usually sugar and/or
starch containing no vitamins or
minerals.

WHY EAT food containing vitamins
and minerals?

To control gum disease

To feel better

To look better

FOODS TO EAT BETWEEN MEALS

THIRSTY: milk, vegetables in form
of juice, fruit juices - frozen or
unsweetened canned

REALLY HUNGRY: Hard boiled eggs,
meat, cheese, nuts

CRUNCHY:
Fresh vegetables: carrots, celery,
cauliflower, etc.

Fresh fruits: oranges, melons,
grapes, etc.

FIG. 6-15. Preventive Measures for Your Dental Health, second sheet (adapted from earlier suggestions by The University of Texas Dental Branch at Houston).

were checked by the patient in completing the questionnaire. Supplements taken by the patient are not included in the evaluation. The third column lists the recommended dietary intake adjusted for that individual and is used for comparison.

Foods High in Essential Nutrients is an information sheet providing the food sources of each nutrient listed in the Dietronics evaluation (Fig. 6-13).

Worksheets for Patient Participation. Preventive Measures for Your Dental Health is a worksheet that becomes a personal account of the patient's dental concern in relationship to the foods he eats, with emphasis placed on those foods that are also food for the bacteria that produce dental disease (Figs. 6-14, 6-15). The important considerations are written on this sheet and are reviewed with the patient. It is personalized by

directly referring to the patient's food intake and food habits, as recorded in his 5-day Food Diary, and the test results.

What Should I Eat? is a list of foods to eat liberally, foods to eat sparingly, and foods to avoid (cariogenic or decay producing) (Figs. 6-16, 6-17). The patient is generally aware of the foods he should be eating but is unaware of the foods that cause decay except perhaps for sugar. Discussing these foods will prevent embarrassment and at the same time prepare the patient so that he can intelligently identify and classify those foods that he has listed in his 5-day Food Diary.

Diet Evaluation is a worksheet in which the patient transposes the foods listed on the 5-day Food Diary into the basic four food groups (Fig. 6-18). The average of each group is computed and compared to the minimum servings suggested. The exercise

WHAT SHOULD I EAT?

FOODS TO EAT LIBERALLY

Eggs:	An average of not less than one a day.
Cheese:	Hard cheese or cottage cheese once a day.
Meat:	Lean meat, poultry, seafoods twice a day.
	One serving liver weekly.
Seafoods:	One serving seafood weekly.

The most desirable methods of cooking these foods are roasted, broiled, baked or stewed. Roasted and broiled meat should be cooked rare or medium rare. Inexpensive cuts of meat are as nutritious as the more expensive cuts.

Milk:	One or two glasses daily – buttermilk, fortified skim, or partially skimmed.

Modern buttermilk and yogurt promote the formation and maintenance of healthy intestinal bacteria.

Fruits:	Two fresh seasonal fruits when available, one being a citrus fruit.

Raw fruits are preferred over cooked or stewed fruits.
Canned fruits should be water packed or no sugar added.

Fruit Juices:	One or two small glasses or one regular glass daily.

Fruit juice is in addition to fresh fruit. It should be a substitute for soft drinks and other beverages. All types of juice are acceptable except those with sugar added. Avoid prune and grape juice as they are high in natural sugars.

Vegetables:	Potatoes plus two other vegetables daily. One should be deep green or yellow.

Potatoes should be baked, boiled or mashed. Avoid fried and chips.
Green vegetables should be string beans, spinach, cauliflower, brussels sprouts, broccoli, cabbage, asparagus, mustard greens.
One raw salad of any kind daily.

Desserts:	Fresh fruits
	Cheese
	Milk puddings occasionally
	Unsweetened gelatin desserts

Gelatin desserts should be made of pure gelatin – no sugar added – with fruit juices and sliced fruit.

FIG. 6-16. What Should I Eat? (adapted from Clark, J. W., Cheraskin, E., and Ringsdorf, W. M.: Diet and the Periodontal Patient. pp. 312–314. Springfield, Ill., Charles C Thomas, 1970).

WHAT SHOULD I EAT?

FOODS TO EAT SPARINGLY

	The amount of these foods eaten by an individual should depend on several factors such as weight and physical activity. The overweight and sedentary person should eat less. The underweight and active person should eat more of these foods.
Bread:	One slice daily not to exceed two slices. Whole grain is preferred. If whole grain cereal is eaten, then one slice of whole grain or high protein bread unless caloric requirements justify more.
Cereals:	Whole grains which require cooking.
Fat:	Where possible use fat of vegetable origin (unsaturated) rather than animal origin (saturated). Vegetable fats should be liquid.
Non-nutrient Dietary Factors:	Artificial sweeteners should be used only in limited amounts. Caffeine-containing foods and drugs should be used sparingly. Examples are: coffee, tea, cola drinks, aspirin, APC, ASA Compound, Cafergot, Coricidin, Empirin Compound, Fiorinal, 4 Way Cold Tablet, Sulfayne, Stanback and Trigesic.

FOODS TO AVOID - CARIOGENIC - DECAY PRODUCING FOODS

Desserts	Crackers	Applesauce
Cake	Pancakes	Apple juice
Cookies	Waffles	Dried fruits
Pies	White bread	Raisins
Coffee cake	Dry cereal	Kool-Aid
Doughnuts	Rice	Carbonated drinks
Custard	Sweet rolls	Chocolate milk
Pudding	Marmalade	Chocolate drinks
Ice milk	Honey	Sauces
Ice cream	Jam	Salad dressings
Sherbets	Jellies	Mayonnaise
Jello	Syrup	Gravy
Chocolate	Catsup	Cream sauces
Candy	Sugar	Canned peas and corn
Chewing gum	Canned fruit	Canned soup
Marshmallows	Frozen fruits	

FIG. 6-17. What Should I Eat? (adapted from Clark, J. W., Cheraskin, E., and Ringsdorf, W. M.: Diet and the Periodontal Patient. pp. 312-314. Springfield, Ill., Charles C Thomas, 1970). Foods to Avoid, courtesy of Dr. Arthur Alban.

Name _____

DIET EVALUATION

FOOD GROUPS			Servings per day						
RECOMMENDED DAILY SERVINGS	FOODS		Day 1	Day 2	Day 3	Day 4	Day 5	Average	What I Need
Milk Group Child – 3 to 4 servings Adolescent – 4 or more Adult – 2 servings	Cheese Ice cream All milks								
Meat Group 2 or more servings	Meat Dry beans Fish Dry peas Eggs Chicken Peanut butter								
Vegetable and Fruit Group 4 or more servings	Citrus fruits Yellow vegetables Dark green vegetables All other fruits and vegetables								
Bread and Cereal Group 4 or more servings	Rice Spaghetti Noodles Crackers Baked products Breakfast cereals Enriched or whole grain breads								

FIG. 6-18. Diet Evaluation (adapted from earlier suggestions by The University of Texas Dental Branch at Houston).

PARTY TIME SNACKS

Eating between meals is not necessarily an undesirable habit. Evidence shows that spreading the daily food intake out over five or six meals helps to stablize the blood sugar, decrease fatigue and prevent obesity. THESE FOODS SHOULD BE TAKEN FROM THE LIST <u>FOODS TO EAT LIBERALLY</u>.

Milk Group
    Milk - skim, whole or buttermilk
        Flavored milk drinks:
        Shake together 1/2 cup orange juice and 1/2 cup cold milk. Pour into chilled glasses.
        Shake together 1/4 cup unsweetened pineapple juice with 1/2 cup cold milk.
        Combine 3/4 cup cold milk, 1/2 cup tomato-vegetable cocktail juice, 1/2 tsp. Worcestershire sauce and salt to taste. Blend. Pour into chilled glasses.
    Cheese - all kinds - cheddar, cottage or cream
        Serve in finger-length sticks of cheddar cheese, swiss or brick.
        Make kabobs by alternating cheese cubes and fruit pieces such as banana, grapes, pineapple, cherries on toothpicks.
        Put walnut or pecan halves together sandwich-style with a soft cheese spread as the filling.
        Cream cheese balls rolled in chopped nuts.
        Cheese Popcorn: Place two quarts popped popcorn in an oven-proof bowl. Dot with 1/4 cup butter. Sprinkle with 1 cup grated cheddar or parmesan cheese and 1 tsp. salt. Heat in oven 300 degrees for 12-15 minutes. Toss well.

Meat Group
    Nuts of all kinds
    Shrimp on toothpicks with tomato cocktail sauce. Shrimp salad placed in the shell of a scooped-out hard roll.
    Deviled eggs
    Sardines, canned salmon or kippered salmon wedges

Vegetable-Fruit Group
    Dip ends of carrot, celery or cucumber sticks into softened cream cheese sprinkled with minced parsley.
    Tomato shell quarters filled with cream cheese filling.
    Peppers - slices or strips
    Apple slices with cheddar cheese
    Pear halves spread with cream cheese and sprinkled with chopped nuts.
    Combine one 3 oz package softened cream cheese and one 2 1/4 oz can deviled ham. Blend. Use to stuff bite size pieces of celery.
    Celery filled with cheese, cottage cheese or peanut butter.

Bread-Cereal Group
    Whole grain bread sandwiches filled with meat, fish or cheese fillings.
    Shredded wheat type crackers
    Place 4 cups ready to eat puffed rice, wheat or corn cereal in baking dish. Heat in oven 350 degrees for 10 minutes. Pour 1/4 cup melted butter over cereal. Salt to taste. Toss well. Serves 8-10 persons.

FIG. 6-19. Party time snacks.

MEAL PLANNING

THE TRADITIONAL THREE MEALS A DAY

The Four Food Groups and the Recommended Number of Servings per day
Milk Group - Adult, two glasses of milk
Meat Group - Two or more servings
Vegetable-Fruit Group - Four or more servings
Bread-Cereal Group - Four or more servings

Breakfast Choices
Fruit or juice - fresh, frozen, canned
Main dish - eggs, beans, fish, poultry
Bread and/or cereal - cereal, biscuits,
  tortillas, toast, cornbread, pancakes
  Use enriched or whole grain products
Beverage - milk, tea or coffee

Lunch Choices
Main dish - soup made with milk or
  vegetables, casserole, sandwich,
  dried beans
Vegetables and/or fruits - fresh, frozen
  or canned fruits, raw vegetables, salads
Bread - sandwiches, crackers, rolls
  Use enriched or whole grain products
Beverage - milk for adults too!

Dinner Choices
Main dish - meat, fish, poultry, eggs,
  cheese or beans. Use liver and organ
  meats often.
Vegetables and/or fruits - Use two
  servings at this meal. A dark green
  or deep yellow every day. Fresh,
  frozen or canned fruit.
Bread - rice, spaghetti, noodles, tortillas,
  that have been enriched, and enriched
  or whole grain bread and rolls
Beverage - milk, tea or coffee
Desserts - fruits, simple puddings, custards

Snack Choices
Select with Care. AVOID SUGAR
Nutritious foods should be considered
a part of the total food requirement for
one day. Select these from milk, cheese,
sandwich fillings, vegetables, fruits,
fruit juices, and nuts. You may wish to
set aside a shelf in the refrigerator or
cupboard with foods to be used for snacks.

SUGGESTED MENUS

Breakfast
Citrus fruit
Eggs - two
Whole wheat toast
Margarine or butter
Milk, tea or coffee

Lunch
Vegetable soup
Tuna fish on whole
  wheat bread
Margarine or butter
Cottage cheese-fruit salad
Milk, tea or coffee

Dinner
Sliced ham
Baked sweet potatoes
French style green beans
Carrot and celery sticks
Whole wheat hard roll
Margarine or butter
Chilled fruit cup for dessert
Milk, tea or coffee

Breakfast
Tomato juice
Cooked cereal
Honey, milk
Applesauce
Milk, tea or coffee

Lunch
Chili with meat
Whole wheat crackers
Carrot and celery sticks
Custard
Milk, tea or coffee

Dinner
Fried chicken
Baked potato with sour cream,
  cheese, onion, bacon bits
Asparagus
Fresh vegetable salad
Hard roll, margarine or butter
Baked apple for dessert
Milk, tea or coffee

FIG. 6-20. Meal planning.

HOW TO HAVE A HAPPY DAY

A TYPICAL AMERICAN BREAKFAST
Fruit or juice which supplies natural sugar. Cereals, pancakes, waffles, coffee cakes, and toast which supply starch which is quickly changed to sugar during digestion. Sugar added to cereal and coffee and jam and jellies.

WHAT THIS MEAL DOES
It rapidly increases the blood sugar causing an outpouring of insulin from the pancreas. This in turn causes the liver and muscles to withdraw more sugar for storage, but as digestion continues, sugar keeps pouring into the blood stream with more insulin being produced. Too much sugar is withdrawn from the blood as the result of this oversupply of insulin. The amount of energy you have is dependent upon the amount of sugar in the blood stream that the cells can draw upon for use. The symptoms of a body deprived of sugar are hunger, craving for sweets, growling of the intestines, slowed thinking, confusion, nerves tense, irritable, grouchy, moody, depressed, tired, headaches, weakness and wobbliness, palpitations, nausea and vomiting, fainting and blackouts.

WHAT TO DO ABOUT IT
Eat a breakfast of low sugar and fat and moderate protein. Digestion will be slower, the sugar will dribble slowly into the blood stream. The pancreas will not overproduce insulin, and you will have a sustained energy hour after hour all day long.

FOODS TO INCLUDE IN AN ENERGY BREAKFAST
Whole milk
Eggs
Ham, sausage, ground beef, fish, chicken
Hot cereals
Fruit
Cottage cheese, other forms of cheese

IF YOU CANNOT EAT IT, DRINK IT
1 glass citrus juice
Eggnog - recipe
    1 egg   1/4 cup pwd skim milk
    1 tsp sugar   1 cup whole milk
    Beat until smooth. Flavor with
    vanilla and nutmeg. Chill

PROTEIN FOODS ARE EXPENSIVE FOODS, BUT THEY WILL HELP SAVE YOUR TEETH and preserve your health.

TO THINK ABOUT
Eat between meals to maintain high blood sugar levels. A suggestion: 1 glass whole
    milk and 100 calories of fresh fruit.
Summer heat decreases the appetite for protein resulting in increased sugared drinks
    and ice cream which in effect decrease the blood sugar. Exercise such as swimming
    uses available sugar in the body producing fatigue and crankiness.
It is felt that virus infections are usually contracted when the blood sugar is extremely low.
Excessive use of coffee, cigarettes and alcohol is related to and lowers the blood sugar.
Hunger occurs when the blood sugar drops to about 70 mg; twelve hours after a typical
    American dinner, the blood sugar is about 95 mg or more.
If you are not hungry in the morning, you may have eaten too much the evening before.

EAT BREAKFAST LIKE A KING, LUNCH LIKE A PRINCE, AND DINNER LIKE A PAUPER

SIZE OF SERVINGS - ADULT
Milk Group - 1 cup milk; Meat Group - 3 oz, average size of hamburger patty, 1 chicken leg; Vegetable-Fruit Group - 1/2 cup; Bread-Cereal Group - 1 slice bread, 1 tortilla, 3/4 cup ready to eat cereal, 1/2 cup cooked cereal, macaroni, spaghetti, rice, grits, or noodles.

FIG. 6-21. How to have a happy day.

TO SAVE DOLLARS

PLAN AHEAD

Take advantage of the weekly specials, locally produced foods, and the plentiful as
well as foods in season. Buy only what is needed to avoid waste and spoilage.
Cook from "scratch."

Use less expensive cuts and grades of meat.

Use dried beans, peas, macaroni products and rice in combination with meat, eggs,
milk, cheese and fish.

In buying eggs, the grade indicates quality. The size indicates weight. Fresh, high
quality eggs (Grade AA or A) may not be the largest. These are preferred for poaching
and frying. Grade B and C may be cheaper and can be used for casseroles, meat
loaves and general cooking. The color of the shell does not affect the nutritive value
of the egg. It may affect the cost.

Use only enriched white bread, macaroni, spaghetti, rice, flour, pancake flour, cakes,
cookies, pies and crackers. Use dark bread labeled 100% whole wheat.

Milk should be fortified with vitamin D. Low fat milk should be fortified with vitamins
A and D. Margarine should be fortified with vitamin A.

Iodized salt should be used to prevent simple goiter.

Use a list to shop. Be flexible. Do not shop when you are hungry. Do not hurry.
Read the labels to determine the best buys in both nutrition and cost. To determine
the best buy, divide the number of servings into the price of the item.

FOOD STORAGE

Meat and poultry - Do not wash. Store in the coldest part of the refrigerator. Cook
within a few days. Ground meat or meat cut in small pieces should be kept very
cold and used within 24 hours.

Bread - Wrap in moisture-resistant material. Store at room temperatures in a clean,
dry, ventilated container or drawer away from heat producing equipment. Dampness
and temperatures above 80 degrees will encourage mold. Bread can be stored in the
refrigerator to prevent mold, but this will hasten staling. Heating stale bread helps
to restore freshness.

Cereal - Keep in tightly covered containers.

Eggs - Store in refrigerator. Egg whites can be stored in tightly covered containers,
egg yolks should be covered with water to prevent drying out.

Cheese - Hard or semi-hard should be kept in a tight container or wrapped in moisture-
proof paper in the refrigerator. Wiping with vinegar will help prevent mold.

Fruits and vegetables - Refrigerate unwashed in crisper pans or plastic bags. Washing
hastens spoilage. Bananas should be kept at room temperatures. These foods
should be washed thoroughly to remove insecticides and herbicides.

Fats - Butter and margarine and open containers of salad dressing should be kept in the
refrigerator.

Coffee, tea and nuts should be stored in the refrigerator when in use.

COOKING

The vitamins and minerals lie just below the skins of some fruits and vegetables. These
foods should be eaten raw, cooked or peeled thinly. Cut vegetables just prior to
cooking or serving to preserve nutrients. Cook quickly in small amounts of water.
Use leftover water for sauces, gravies, etc.

Use low or moderate heat for cooking all meats to reduce shrinkage, drying, and to
preserve the juices.

Avoid leftovers - Nutrients are removed each time the food is reheated.

FIG. 6-22. To Save Dollars.

HAPPY BIRTHDAY SUGGESTIONS

Nutritious Beverages:
   Serve in paper cups or small individual cartons. Use colorful straws.
   Types of drink - milk, tomato juice, the unsweetened fruit juices such as orange,
      grapefruit, grape or pineapple.
   Freeze fruit juices in ice cube trays and serve in glasses of juice.

Finger Foods:
   Raw vegetables - carrots, celery, radishes, tomato, cabbage and lettuce wedges,
      cucumber rings, cauliflower flowerettes.
   Fruits wrapped in cellophane - apples, bananas, peaches, plums, grapes, bing
      cherries, tangerines, pears or strawberries. "Boats" of orange wedges with
      toothpicks as masts and small pieces of paper as sails.
   Cheese and meat cubes and shrimp speared with colored toothpicks. Serve with
      crackers.
   Celery stuffed with cheese, cottage cheese or peanut butter.
   Hard cooked eggs, deviled eggs.
   Cheese dips with vegetable sticks.
   Peanuts, popcorn or potato chips in individual packages.
   Treasure Logs - cut thin slices of lean beef or ham. In each slice, roll a piece
      of mild flavored cheese.
   Cream Cheese Balls - soften cream cheese, add mustard and minced parsley.
      Roll in small balls and then in chopped nuts.
   Animal Shaped Cheese - cut American cheese or any hard cheese with a cookie
      cutter into desired shapes.

Sandwiches:
   Cut bread into unusual shapes with cookie cutters. Make faces or other designs
      with raisins, carrot curls, sliced olives or nuts.
   Favorite spreads are egg, meat or fish plain or in combination with cheese.

Birthday Cakes:
   Cut an unsliced loaf of day old bread the long way into three or four slices. Use
      two or three different kinds of egg, meat or cheese spreads between layers and
      frost the outside with cream cheese (tinted if you like). Place candles on top.
      Slice the loaf into ribbons when the children are ready to eat.

   Add 1 cup sliced or diced fresh fruit (banana, apples, peaches, pears, grapes, etc.)
      to 2 cups stiffly whipped cream. Fold together. Pour into glass pie or cake pan.
      Decorate with candles. After candles are blown out, dish into individual dishes.
      This may be frozen if appropriate fruit is used.

Ice Cream:
   3 eggs   1 1/2 cups milk   1 1/2 cups cream   1/2 teaspoon salt
   3/4 cup sugar   1 tablespoon flour   2 teaspoons vanilla
   Heat milk in double boiler. Beat egg yolks until thick and add 1/2 cup sugar and
   flour. Beat until thick and smooth. Add to heated milk and cook until thick. Cool
   and chill. Beat egg whites stiff but not dry. Add 1/4 cup sugar. Fold into chilled
   custard. Whip cream and add to custard, add vanilla. Pour into refrigerator trays.
   Stir 2 or 3 times while freezing.

FIG. 6-23. Happy Birthday Suggestions.

CHILDREN

SIZE OF SERVINGS

Food	Ages 2-3 years	Ages 4-6 years
Milk _____	1/2 to 1 cup	3/4 to 1 cup
Meat, fish, poultry, cottage cheese, cheese ____	3 tablespoons	4 tablespoons
Egg _____	1 whole	1 whole
Potato _____	1-2 tablespoons	4 tablespoons
Vegetable - raw _____	2-3 small pieces	3-4 small pieces
cooked _____	1-2 tablespoons	2-4 tablespoons
Fruit, canned or fresh _____	1/3 cup	1/2 cup
Citrus fruit and juice _____	1/4 to 1/3 cup	1/3 to 2/3 cup
Bread _____	1/2 slice	1 slice
Cereal - ready to eat _____	1/3 cup	1/2 cup
cooked _____	2 tablespoons	1/4 cup

SMALL SERVINGS are a must. A large serving may discourage the child.

THE CHILD WHO DOES NOT LIKE MILK to drink: Make cereals, soups and desserts with milk. Serve cheese, cottage cheese and ice cream. The foods that contain calcium are cheese, milk, nuts, dried figs, dried beans and dried peas, dark green leafy vegetables such as dandelion greens, mustard and turnip greens, collards, kale and broccoli.

FOR THE HIGH-STRUNG, EMOTIONAL AND PRE-ADOLESCENT CHILD, a child craving sweets, serve more protein in the diet. These same foods will also be high in the vitamin B complex. Serve ground meat for the very young, mild flavored fish such as haddock, halibut, tuna, salmon, cottage cheese, peanut butter, dried beans and dried peas, milk, eggs, custards and scramble egg sandwiches. A diet high in protein reduces the desire or craving for sweets.

TO HELP INSURE A "HAPPY CHILD" AND "HAPPY PARENTS," think about the following:
Rest - A tired or excited child cannot enjoy his food. Allow a quiet time before meals so he can "slow down."
Attractive Food - How the food looks, tastes and feels in the mouth is important to the child. He likes the bright color of food such as green peas or red tomatoes. He likes colorful plates, cups and place mats. He prefers mild flavors of carrots, new potatoes, custards and bananas. The textures he prefers are moisture in meat and eggs, smoothness of milk soups and puddings and the crispness of raw fruits and vegetables. He does not like his food mixed. He wants to be able to identify the food.
New Food - Offer only one new food at a time. Let the child see you eat and enjoy it. Expect him to like it too. Be casual about new foods. Avoid forcing the food or making a fuss about it.
Please the child occasionally with his favorite food. By pleasing him, he will want to please you.
Desserts should be served casually as the usual part of the meal. Do not make them seem more desirable than other food. Offer wholesome desserts such as custards, milk puddings and fruit. Pies and cakes, etc., are less nutritious and can be served occasionally.
Let the child set the table, serve his own food, pour his own milk when he is able and prepare food. These will increase his interest and improve his eating habits. Relax Parents - Have meal time a happy family affair. Do not worry about THE WHAT, THE HOW MUCH, or THE HOW he eats. When parents stop worrying children start eating.

FIG. 6-24. Children, an information sheet dealing with feeding difficulties.

NUTRITIONAL RECORD

Name _____ Date _____ Chart # _____
Height _____ Weight _____ Sex _____ Age _____
Grade at school _____ Employment _____ Hours _____
Father's occupation _____ Mother's occupation _____
Family members and ages: Boys _____ Girls _____
Child care: Home _____ School _____ Elsewhere _____

SECTION I - EATING PATTERN
Meals eaten at home _____ Restaurant _____ Elsewhere _____
Who plans and prepares meals _____
Time awaken _____ Breakfast _____
A.M. snacks _____ Lunch _____
Afternoon snacks _____
Dinner _____
Bedtime snacks _____ Bedtime hour _____
Remarks _____

SECTION II - FOOD SELECTION
Type of diet _____
Foods influenced by religious beliefs _____
Foods influenced by ethnic affiliation _____
Specific foods eaten daily _____ time _____
Reason _____
Craving for specific foods _____
Dietary supplements being taken _____
Suggested dietary supplements - Dietronics _____
Remarks _____

SECTION III - NUTRITIONAL EVALUATION - DIETRONICS

Nutrients	%RDA	Amount		Nutrients	%RDA	Amount	
Protein			gm	Calcium			mg
Calories				Magnesium			mg
Carbohydrates			gm	Phosphorus			mg
Sugar			tsps	Iron			mg
Vitamin A			USPU	Rcal/Cal			
Vitamin E			I.U.	Calc/Phos			
Vitamin B-1			mg	Equivalent to calories _____ tsps sugar			
Vitamin B-2			mg	Cereal			
Niacin			mg	Protein			
Vitamin B-6			mg	Veg.- Fruit			
Pantothenic Acid			mg	Dairy			
Vitamin B-12			mcg	Plaque forming foods			
Vitamin C			mg	Nonplaque forming foods			

SECTION IV
Five Day Food Diary indicates a typical week _____ Reason _____
Number of servings from the Four Food Groups as determined from the Five Day Food
Diary: Milk _____ Meat _____ Vegetables and Fruits _____
Bread and Cereal _____

FIG. 6-25. Nutritional Record.

is completed by the patient himself as he suggests the foods he can eat or omit to improve his food selection. He becomes aware of the groups of foods he is eating as well as diet inadequacies.

If Dietronics or a similar service is not used, then the accuracy of this exercise is of the utmost importance and the interpretation of its results should be carefully considered. What may seem an optimum selection of food for the one week is in reality a deficient diet; for example, the table below is the record of a 61-year-old woman. The example

5-Day Food Diary	Recommended	Dietronics
0.4	Milk 2	1.1
2.8	Protein 2	1.4
3.2	Fruits and vegetables 4	1.5
3.0	Bread and cereal 4	1.4

compares the average number of servings in the basic four food groups. Further discussion with the patient indicated that the Dietronics evaluation is more accurate over a longer time than that recorded for the 5-day period.

Informational Sheets. These are designed to meet the specific needs of the patient. Party Time Snacks (Fig. 6-19) is a listing of nutritious between-meal or party time refreshments according to their placement within the four food groups. Meal Planning (Fig. 6-20) lists food choices for breakfast, lunch, dinner, and snacks as well as suggested menus for 2 days. Patients appreciate menu ideas. How to Have a Happy Day (Fig. 6-21) stresses the need for eating a protein breakfast. It is related to a simple discussion of low blood sugar and the body's need for nutrients even in the heat of summertime.

To Save Dollars (Fig. 6-22) suggests ways to save money yet eat nutritious foods. Happy Birthday Suggestions (Fig. 6-23) is a paper prepared for the family with small children. It provides suggestions for party refreshments and includes several recipe ideas. The information sheet, Children (Fig.

6-24), is directed primarily to the difficulties encountered in the feeding of some children. Many children do not like milk. This is a real concern to mothers.

These fact sheets do not solve all problems for all patients. Their purpose is to assist the patient in difficult situations. They extend to the patient a sympathetic, understanding, and helpful hand.

The Nutritional Record and Its Significance. For effective nutritional counseling, the control therapist must be aware of certain personal habits of the patient that relate to food selection and eating habits. The Nutritional Record (Fig. 6-25) provides an opportunity to obtain this information, usually through direct discussion.

In the statistical portion of the form, the height, weight, sex, age, occupation, working hours, and family members relate to the amount of nutrients required by the individual, to the food selections, and to the eating pattern.

Section I deals with the eating patterns. Meals eaten at restaurants can be less nutritious than those prepared and served at home because of the time between preparation and consumption and the extensive use of leftovers. The person who plans and prepares the meals may not be the mother. It may be the oldest daughter or even the son. The daily routine indicates the eating habits of the patient and points to areas for improvement.

Section II, food selection, provides the *why* certain foods are eaten. It may be indicative of physical or emotional disturbances and cultural or religious beliefs.

Section III and IV are for recording the nutritional evaluation–Dietronics and the servings in the basic four food groups.

All these factors are taken into consideration as plans and constructive nutritional discussion are carried out with the patient.

Personal Dental Profile. This profile (Fig. 6-26) provides a summary of the oral and nutritional conditions that relate to the patient's dental disease. The Oral Conditions review the signs and symptoms present

PERSONAL DENTAL PROFILE

Name _____   Date _____

Oral Conditions	Unfavorable	Favorable
Plaque Index _____	4 3 2 1	0
Gum tissue _____	Bleeding, puffy, tender	Firm, stippled, no bleeding
Decay _____	Cavities	No cavities
Bone loss _____	Pockets _____	No pockets
Microscopic bacterial examination _____	Well organized, massive	Few bacteria

Test Results		
Plaque - D-K Test _____	+4 +3 +2	+1 -1
Saliva		
Flow - unstimulated _____	_____	3.7 ml average young adult
stimulated _____	Less than 8.0 ml	13.8 ml average young adult
Viscosity _____	2.0 minutes or over _____	1.3-1.4 minutes _____
Acid Buffering Capacity _____	4 5 6 drops	7 8 9 10-14 drops
Bacterial Activity		
Snyder Test _____	4+ 3+ 2+	1+ negative
Alkaline Phosphatase _____	Active, highly active	Inactive
Acid Phosphatase _____	Moderate, highly active	Inactive

Nutritional Factors		
Oral Glucose Clearance Test _____	25-30 minutes _____	Short period of time _____
Lingual Ascorbic Acid Test - Vitamin C _____	Over 20 seconds _____	Less than 15 seconds _____
Daily Recommended Requirement Calcium _____	_____	_____
Daily Recommended Requirement Phosphorus _____		
Percent of calories from refined carbohydrates _____	15% and up _____	15% and less _____
Number of teaspoons of sugar eaten per day _____		As few as possible _____
Average daily exposures to plaque forming foods _____	_____	As few as possible _____
Average daily exposures to nonplaque forming foods ___		As many as possible _____
Average daily servings Four Food Groups		
Cereal _____	_____	4 minimum _____
Protein _____	_____	2 minimum _____
Vegetable - Fruit _____	_____	4 minimum _____
Dairy _____	_____	2 minimum _____

NUTRIENT DEFICIENCIES   FOOD PRESCRIPTION   COMMENTS

FIG. 6-26. Personal Dental Profile.

at the first disease control session that are primarily treated with oral hygiene procedures. The Test Results are correlated to provide more significance and understanding of the oral conditions. The Nutritional Factors are summarized and related to specific oral conditions as well as to the test results. The Food Prescription space on the dental profile is for listing foods that should be added to the diet to bring it up to adequacy.

Disease Control Family Summary. When two or more members of the same family go through the control program, a family summary is prepared (Fig. 6-27). This summary lists the test results for all members as well as the appointments remaining in the program.

SUMMARY

It may be hard for some to associate dental health with what a person eats for breakfast, lunch, and dinner. Diet evaluation is a health service that is not readily available to the public. If dentistry is willing to make the effort, the best interests of dentistry will be served and a real and lasting service will be rendered. It must be properly presented so that the patient's needs will be filled and assistance given so that he can carry out and achieve actual results. Treating the total individual is to provide nutritional counseling on what to eat rather than just what not to eat.

Many factors enter into dental disease, and an effort should be directed toward the total problem and not just a segment of its cause. The variability of different patients in their response to disease is due in large part to the ability of the body to withstand infection or to its lack of power to combat the insults that it receives.

The purpose of nutritional counseling is to enable the patient to better understand

DISEASE CONTROL FAMILY SUMMARY

Family Member	Vitamin C Test	Saliva Tests	Nutritional Evaluation	Comments	Remain. Appts.
	Date	Date	Date		
	Date	Date	Date		
	Date	Date	Date		
	Date	Date	Date		
	Date	Date	Date		
	Date	Date	Date		
	Date	Date	Date		

FIG. 6-27. Disease Control Family Summary.

and appreciate the food he eats. A choice has to be made in food selection, and with a conscious effort, decisions can be made to provide protection as well as nourishment to the body.

Seemingly few patients are informed on the subject of nutrition. It is practical information that children as well as adults can benefit from. It is the patient's interest in and his appreciation for nutritional counseling that will insure the continuation of this service in the dental office.

PART III
The Procedures

The awareness of clinical and educational
needs of the dental patient is established
through progressive steps that include
the exchange of philosophies, establishment
of priorities, and mutual trust and understanding.

Presenting Disease Control

The future is bringing with it expanded duties of the auxiliaries, resulting in less "doctor time" spent with the patient. To effectively motivate patients to control their dental disease, the dentist must give more time.

Dental education in the past has failed. The dental education of a preventive dental practice will succeed if the dentist takes the time to communicate with the patient. The thorough examination is the beginning step in this path to success. If, instead of delegating the duty, the doctor takes the time himself to communicate the need for the control of oral disease, the patient will respond with action. "If the doctor thinks my bleeding gums are serious and I should learn to prevent it, I will." It is as simple as this.

The dentist, after having taken the patient through the first part of the visit 1 of disease control, can delegate to the control therapist the remaining duties of teaching the why.

THE THREE-PHASE EXAMINATION FOR THE ADULT

The three-phase examination for the adult requires three appointments. The procedure followed closely parallels that suggested by Dr. Robert Barkley.

Phase I

Time allowed for appointment: 30 minutes

1. With the patient's arrival, the dentist is notified by means of the Valcom signal system.
2. The receptionist Check List is completed through Appointment scheduled (see Fig. 3-2).
3. Using the Phase I Examination Check List (Fig. 7-1), the receptionist completes her observations, takes the medical history, and obtains the name and address of the patient's physician.
4. The *Welcome to Our Office* is given to the patient to read in the reception room prior to being seen by the dentist (see Fig. 3-4).

Equipment for the examination in the operatory:

Basic tray setup:
  Mouth mirror
  Explorer no. 23
  Cotton pliers
  Evacuator tip
  2-by-2-inch gauze
Patient's chest towel
Impression trays
Modified Snyder test

Procedure:

1. The chair-side assistant places the towel on the patient and indicates to the dentist through the signal system that the patient is seated and ready.
2. The dentist enters, introduces himself, and asks how he can be of help.
3. The chair-side assistant records the remarks of the patient as the dentist asks

PHASE I
EXAMINATION CHECK LIST

Name _____ Date _____ Chart # _____

Receptionist's Observations:
    Initial request to Receptionist _____
    Spontaneous comments about health _____
    Immediate problems to be cared for _____
    Attitude: Circle one   Enthusiastic   Cooperative   Skeptical
    Fears or dislikes mentioned _____

Medical History taken by Receptionist
                          Date of birth _____
    Do you have any history of heart disease? _____ Rheumatic Fever _____
    Do you have diabetes? _____ How well controlled? _____
    Do you have any history of kidney or liver disease? _____
    Do you have excessive bleeding? _____
    Have you recently had a serious illness? _____
    Have you recently had excessive emotional stress? _____
    Have you ever had radiation treatments? _____ Date _____
    Are you allergic to drugs? _____
    Are you taking any medications? _____

Physician's Name _____ Date of last visit _____
Address _____
        _____

Dentist's Observations:
    How can I help you? _____
    Patient's response to explanation of diagnostic procedures _____
    Age of first dental appointment _____ Any unpleasant dental experiences? _____
    Was care regular? _____ How much care was needed? _____
    What are/were parents' dental conditions and care habits? _____
    _____
    Any edentulous? _____
    What are/were brothers'-sisters' dental conditions and care habits? _____
    _____
    Any edentulous? _____
    What is/was spouse's dental condition and care habits? _____
    _____
    Any edentulous? _____
    What are/were the children's dental conditions and care habits? _____
    _____
    How would you describe your present dental health?   Good   Fair   Poor
    What type of dental care have you received within the past five years? _____
    _____
    Do you think your dental disease is active or controlled? _____
    Have you ever been taught to control it? _____
    How do you feel about losing your teeth? _____

Obtain full series x-rays, apical and bite wing.   Obtain impressions for study models
Obtain centric relation records   Obtain Snyder Test
Obtain picture, if desired

FIG. 7-1. Phase I Examination Check List (adapted from Dr. Robert Barkley).

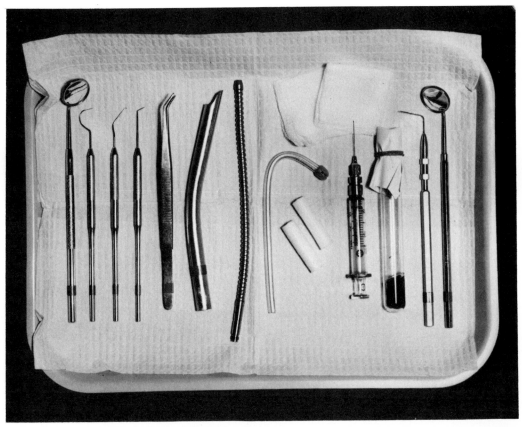

FIG. 7-2. Tray setup for Phase II of the dental examination.

the questions outlined in Dentist's Observations on the Examination Check List. The format is memorized by the dentist and the questions and answers are in the form of conversation.

4. The chair-side assistant has the patient drool saliva into a test tube containing Snyder medium, for the modified Snyder test.

5. A complete oral x-ray series is taken.

6. Impressions for diagnostic models are taken and the centric relation recorded.

7. A Polaroid picture is taken, if desired by the dentist.

8. The post-treatment information messages on full survey of x-rays and diagnostic models are given to the patient and reviewed with him by the chair-side assistant.

9. The patient is dismissed to the receptionist who makes an appointment for Phase II to follow 2 to 4 days later.

The receptionist prepares a letter to the patient's physician for the patient to sign at Phase II (see Fig. 3-16).

Phase II

Time allowed for appointment: 30 minutes
Equipment:
Oral examination tray setup (Fig. 7-2):
　Two mouth mirrors
　Three explorers—No. 17, 23, 6
　Cotton pliers
　Evacuator tip and saliva ejector
　BioLite transilluminator
　Hu-Friedy periodontal pocket probe
　Two 2-by-2-inch gauze strips
　Two cotton rolls
　Lingual ascorbic acid test (Pro-C test)
　Snyder medium if necessary
Patient's models mounted on the articulator
Patient's x-rays mounted on the view box
　(Fig. 7-3)

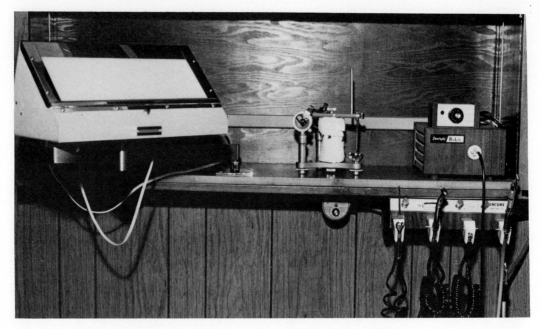

FIG. 7-3. X-ray view box and diagnostic models.

The Chart:

The Examination Check List (Figs. 7-4, 7-5) consists of two pages. It includes findings concerning the diagnostic models, the x-rays, occlusion, intraoral inspection, and a listing of tests to be conducted. It concludes with the patient's concerns and attitudes.

The findings are tabulated on the third page of the examination chart (Fig. 7-6). This is used to summarize and record the conditions in the mouth as they are observed by the dentist; his comments are recorded by the chair-side assistant. Treatment recommendations are also noted.

A fourth page of the chart, Confidential Remarks (Fig. 7-7), is provided for use by all staff members for recording information relating to cancelled appointments, dissatisfactions, or any negative data. Specific treatment is not recorded on this form.

Procedure:

1. The chair-side assistant seats and places the chest towel on the patient.

2. The chair-side assistant gives the patient his models to observe. She records any pertinent remarks on the chart.

3. The chair-side assistant indicates to the dentist (signal system) that the patient is ready.

4. The dentist and the patient observe together the patient's models and answer questions dictated by the chair-side assistant as she follows the check list.

5. The examination Check List is completed.
   a. Concerning the models
   b. Concerning the x-ray findings
   c. Intraoral inspection

6. BioLite transillumination examination is completed and recorded on the chart after location of cavities on the Examination Check List.

7. Lingual ascorbic acid test is taken.

8. The patient's attitude and comments are recorded.

9. The post-treatment information sheet on oral examination is given to the patient and briefly reviewed with him.

10. The patient is dismissed to the receptionist.

PHASE II

EXAMINATION CHECK LIST

Name _____ Date _____ Chart # _____

Models
    Any missing teeth? - Chart
    Position of remaining teeth _____
    Any disfigurement of anterior teeth? _____
    Are the anterior teeth being bruxed? _____
    Any loss of papillae? _____
    Any generalized recession? _____
    Any erosion? - Chart
    Any broken fillings? - Chart
    How are the margins of old fillings? _____
    Occlusal interferences
        Centric _____
        Left lateral _____
        Right lateral _____
    Any potential cusp fracture areas? - Chart
    Any food impaction sites? - Chart
    Any unmanageable bacterial traps? - Chart

X-ray Findings
    Prevalence of fillings: Circle one   Few   Moderate   Many
    Any overhanging margins? - Chart
    Any recurrent cavities? - Chart
    Any new cavities? - Chart
    Any possible pulp infections? - Chart
    Any periapical infections? - Chart
    Any bone loss? - Chart
      Horizontal bone loss - Chart
      Angular bone loss - Chart
    Any widened periodontal membranes? - Chart
    General appearance of supporting tissues _____
    _____
    Any unerupted teeth? - Chart

Occlusion
    Condition of the temporomandibular joint:
    Any popping or clicking?_____
    Any history of popping or clicking?_____
    Any history of pain? _____
    Verify any premature interferences in terminal hinge:
    First prematurity Right _____ Left _____ mm _____
    Verify any skid or deviation _____
    Verify any balancing interferences
    Right lateral _____   Left lateral _____

FIG. 7-4. Phase II Examination Check List (adapted from Dr. Robert Barkley).

PHASE II Examination Check List (continued)

Intraoral Inspection
    Lips _____
    Buccal mucosa _____
    Palate _____
    Floor of mouth _____
    Tongue _____
    Tongue swallow pattern _____
    Oropharynx _____
    Submaxillary areas:
        Lymph nodes _____
        Salivary glands _____
    Periodontal tissue:
        Color of gingival tissue _____
        State of sulcular epithelium _____
        Any pocket formation? - Chart in mm and areas
        Periodontal disease: Circle one Very active Active Limited Very limited
        Need for water spray _____
        Any unmanageable teeth? - Chart
    General appearance of the teeth:
        Are the anterior teeth discolored? _____
        Are the anterior teeth abraded? _____
        Are there spaces between the anterior teeth? ___
        Are the anterior teeth crowded? _____
    General condition of the teeth:
        Oral Hygiene Evaluation: Excellent - 0 Good - 1 Fair - 2 Poor - 3
        Any areas of heavy bacterial accumulation? - Chart
        Amount of calculus _____
        Present restorations and locations - Chart
        Location of cavities - Chart
    State of bacterial control _____
    State of disease manageability _____
Lingual Ascorbic Acid Test _____ seconds
Caries Activities _____
Snyder Test _____
Patient's attitude during examination: Circle one Interested Casual Disinterested
Fears and dislikes of potential treatment possibilities _____

Hopes and desires about future dentistry _____

FIG. 7-5. Continuation of Phase II Examination Check List (adapted from Dr. Robert Barkley).

The patient reads and signs the physician's letter and an appointment is made for 2 to 4 days later for Phase III. Sufficient time should be allowed to prepare the written diagnosis.

Phase III

Time allowed for appointment: 30 minutes (15 minutes for the dentist)

Upon arrival at the office, the patient is given his written diagnosis and is invited to read it in the reception room. (It is necessary to affirm that the patient can read.) A pencil is provided so that he can write down any questions that he may have concerning his diagnosis. Approximately 15 minutes is allowed for this.

Written Diagnosis:

The written diagnosis should reflect the personality and the philosophy of the dentist. A suggested outline follows:

Title

Patient's name and address; date

The Introduction: A statement of philosophy and purpose (Barkley)

The present oral conditions are stated:

Oral environment based on the Snyder test (Sims)

Vitamin C status commentary (Mittelman)

Missing teeth

Location of remaining teeth

Periodontal condition

Cavities

Mouth infections

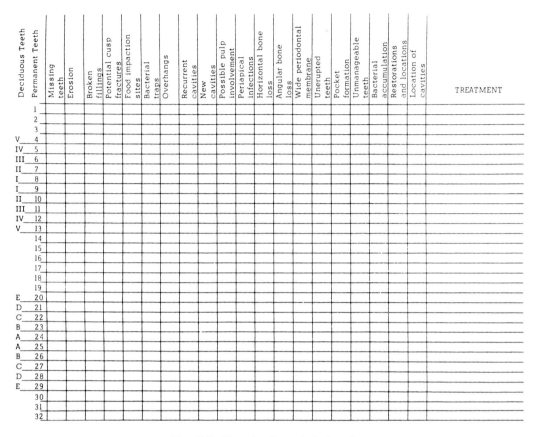

Fig. 7-6. Examination tabulation chart.

Occlusion
Appearance
Oral hygiene evaluation

Treatment recommendations:
   Control dental disease
   Clean the teeth
   Apply fluoride
   Treatment
      Restorations
      Replacement

Limitations of treatment:
   This explains the prognosis that can be
expected with the continuation of present oral conditions, how the patient
can cooperate to change the situation,
and the benefit of controlling dental
disease and of restorative treatment.
The Consultation. Two chairs are made
available in the consultation area of the office.

In the office described in this text, the
Dentist and patient sit on stools in dental
operatory no. 1. Phase II of the dental
examination was conducted in this room at
the last appointment, and the room will
again be used for the next appointment
(disease control visit 1, Part A).

The receptionist escorts the patient into
the area selected for the conference and indicates to the dentist (Valcom signal system)
that the patient is ready.

The dentist and the patient discuss those
points that the patient wishes to review. It
requires very little in the way of explanation,
for the patient has evaluated the situation in
Phase II of the examination and has said in
his own words or agreed that it is sensible
and logical to control his own disease. This
meeting reaffirms his intentions and answers
any questions that he might have.

The conversation varies, but it may be similar to this:

Dentist: Do you have any questions after reading your diagnosis?

Patient: No, but I thought I had been taking care of my teeth just fine all these years.

Dentist: Yes, I know. We now know more about the control of dental disease and are able to pass this information along to you.

After controlling this disease, you will be able to know the difference it makes. From our last conversation and going through the examination procedure, do you have a feeling for your needs?

Patient: Yes. I really would like to have those bridges.

Dentist: Fine, after you and I know that your gums are healed and not puffy and

CONFIDENTIAL REMARKS

Name _____

Date	Remarks

FIG. 7-7. Confidential Remarks portion of chart.

swollen we can go ahead and place those bridges.

The patient acknowledges agreement and acceptance.

Dentist: Nancy will make an appointment for you. Thank you, Bob.

Upon completion of the discussion, the dentist escorts the patient to the business office where the receptionist makes appointments for the disease control program. Financial arrangements are made with the patient, if he desires; otherwise, they are made on the visit in which the prophylaxis and fluoride treatment are performed.

The receptionist makes appointments for the first five visits in the disease control program so that they will fall within a period of 7 to 10 days.

A receipt for the diagnosis is given to the patient.

THE TWO-PHASE EXAMINATION FOR THE CHILD

Phase I

Time allowed for appointment: 30 minutes

If this is the child's first visit to the dentist, the pamphlet *Your Child's First Visit* (ADA) was given or mailed to the parent at the time the appointment was made.

The child arrives and is greeted by the receptionist who signals the dentist of his arrival. The health history (PBP form 91) is completed by the mother in the reception room.

The child enters into the operatory without the mother. The examination, Snyder test, lingual ascorbic acid test, x-rays and impressions for diagnostic models are taken and a photograph if desired by the dentist.

The chart consists of the Child's Examination form (Fig. 7-8), tabulation chart (Fig.

THE CHILD'S EXAMINATION

Name _____ Date _____ Chart # _____

Date of birth _____

PHASE I
    Take Snyder Test _____   Results _____
    Take Vitamin C Test _____   Results _____

    Visual Examination
      Follow chart listing

    Closed Examination of occlusion
      Overbite _____   Overjet _____
      Any crossbites ?
        Posterior: Right _____ Left _____
        Incisor crossbite _____
      Anterior open bite _____
        Tongue thrust _____
        Thumb sucking _____
      Midline discrepancy _____
      Facial asymmetry _____

    Periodontal Disease
      Gingivitis _____   Advanced _____

    Need orthodontic treatment _____

    X-rays taken _____
    Followed by recording on the chart

PHASE II
    Consultation
    Establishing the parent's preventive philosophy

FIG. 7-8. The Child's Examination form. The visual examination follows the examination tabulation chart's listings (Fig. 7-6).

7-6), and the Confidential Remarks part of the adult examination chart (Fig. 7-7).

The mother is given the post-treatment information messages of the procedures carried out for the child and is scheduled for the diagnosis. The patient is included in the diagnosis if he or the dentist so desires.

Phase II

Time allowed for the appointment: 30 minutes

The doctor is notified by signal of the arrival of the parent or parents. The parent and dentist review the x-ray findings. The preventive philosophy is discussed and conclusions arrived at. The treatment plan is determined and questions answered.

The child is scheduled for disease control unless immediate treatment is necessary. Parent and child are scheduled for disease control if the child is very young (see Scheduling for the Control Program, Chapter 3).

THE VARIATION IN NEEDS

The need of the patient takes precedence over procedure. The emergency is treated before examination. The disease control program may be indicated treatment for the emergency patient.

Referrals are accepted for disease control. They are handled the same as any patient going onto the control program.

DISEASE CONTROL
Visit 1, Part A

This patient realizes his need for controlling his disease, but how it will be accomplished is still a mystery to him. The dental examination has demonstrated the signs and symptoms of dental disease to the patient before this appointment.

Time allowed for appointment: 30 minutes productive time and 10 minutes to view the filmstrip

Place: Disease control operatory

Persons involved: Dentist, Certified Dental Assistant, and the patient

The dentist is assisted in the dental operatory by the chair-side assistant, which indirectly informs the patient that she is also capable of presenting the control program. At times she will indeed be called upon to conduct the control sessions in place of the control therapist, and this helps to make the transition from one auxiliary to the other easier and more acceptable to the patient. As a general rule, one auxiliary is responsible for the same patient throughout the entire control program.

Equipment:

Disease control tray setup (Fig. 7-9):
    Patient's chest towel and neck clip
    Mouth mirror
    Explorer
    Cotton pliers
    Straight scaler
    Vacudent tip
    Glass slide and coverslip
    Two 2-by-2-inch gauze strips
    Borofax
    Disclosing tablet
    Unwaxed dental floss
    Bridge threader, if necessary
    Lingual ascorbic acid test, if this was not taken on a previous visit
    Modified Snyder medium, if this test was not taken on a previous visit
    Patient's hand mirror
    Stop watch
    Patient's chart including the Test record (see Fig. 4-6).
    Distilled water for preparation of the slide
    Phase microscope
    Filmstrip *Secrets of the Little World* or *How to Stop Dental Disease*

Procedure:

1. The patient is seated and the chest towel placed.
2. A tube of modified Snyder medium is inoculated if this was not done on a previous visit.
3. The dentist discusses with the patient the mechanism of dental disease.

It is not intended or desired that this discussion take on a passive listening and observing attitude, but rather that a personal involvement will develop and move the patient to action. The discussion of dental disease is actually a breaking down of the

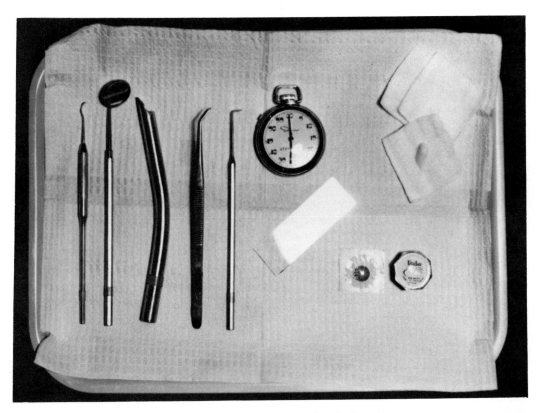

FIG. 7-9. Tray for disease control visit 1, Part A.

barriers of communication that exist between the dentist and the patient. What is said to the patient at this time is not of major concern, but the way in which it is said is of the utmost importance. It is designed to catch the attention and raise the awareness of the patient. There are many reasons a patient will not receive what is being said. The information that he needs will be repeated several times in different ways throughout the program. During one of these presentations the patient will be ready for or the approach will be such that he can understand and believe that which is relevant to him.

A presentation to an adult:

"Today we will be discussing dental disease —the decay of the teeth and the deterioration of the gum and bone around the teeth. It happens to be the number one disease in our population and is more widespread than the common cold. Four out of five children have bleeding gums and nine out of ten adults have gum disease in some form. Mankind has been afflicted and troubled for centuries and it is about time that we do something about it.

"The problem is created because bacteria are present in great numbers in the mouth, and they organize to form what we call the dental plaque. Everything has a name, and this is what it is most frequently called. Another name perhaps more descriptive is the term *microbiota*, meaning "little world." This is appropriate because the organized mass or clump of germs that attaches to the hard structures in the mouth is like many different races living together.

"Bacteria eat the same food that we do, and they are especially fond of sugar. From this they produce energy to live by as well as to form a protective coating called dextran that covers them. This substance is sticky, and not only does it provide protection and storage of food but it helps the bacteria to stick to the teeth, fillings, partials, and dentures. This adhesive quality is needed to isolate and maintain a favorable environment for the bacteria because they do not live or function very well in the saliva.

"Waste products are produced as the end product of the energy cycle derived from the food that they receive. It is these wastes or toxins, which are acid, that cause the teeth to decay. This process takes time, but the destruction of the teeth is accelerated by the frequency and the amount of sugar that is eaten. The more sugar eaten, the more acid that is formed. The more times that sugar is taken into the mouth the more times the acid is able to attack the tooth structure.

"In gum disease, bacteria are present also, but their food is supplied more directly from the gum itself. The toxins that are produced by the bacteria take the skin off the gums, and the bleeding that takes place supplies the germs with their food. This is a never-ending cycle because the more food they get from the gum tissue the more able they are to support themselves and to produce toxins, and thus the conditions remain favorable for their growth. When this happens, it is very much like having the bacteria living inside the body rather than just present in the mouth.

"It is the living bacteria that produce disease. The calculus that forms is mineralized, dead, solidified, plaque material. It does form a dam, allowing the pooling of bacteria, waste products, dead tissue cells, and dead bacteria to build up.

"The weak link in dental disease is that the bacterial plaque can be disorganized and that it takes 24 hours for the bacteria to regroup. Brushing alone does not break the bacterial plaque sufficiently apart between the teeth and under the gum, and this is where most of the problem exists.

"Flossing in a manner that breaks up or disorganizes these bacteria has been developed. Effective results have been accomplished through complete, thorough, once-a-day cleaning of the mouth. The proof is when the teeth and the mouth feel better,

look better, taste better, and smell better. The bleeding of the gums, which is an indicator of gum disease, is stopped in 5 or 6 days. This is a "now" type of thing. A person doesn't have to wait forever to know if he is achieving results. This is important because it is this motivation that helps you to continue to establish the once-daily habit to control and prevent dental disease."

Different age groups require a modification of the story to arouse their interest. Teenagers may relate better to comparing dental disease to ecology, overpopulation, and pollution. Smaller children require a question-and-answer type of format to bring out the points of what dental disease is and why it occurs. The questions from the patient will influence the information, and it becomes personalized to their needs and the conditions that are within their own personal experiences. The placement of emphasis on aspects that relate to the person changes the discussion to conversation rather than a lecture. The matter-of-fact method is not to degrade or turn the patient off but to stimulate interest and the excitement of knowing.

4. The lingual ascorbic acid test is conducted by the dentist if it was not done on a previous visit. The results are discussed with the patient at this time.

5. The dentist procures plaque from the lingual or distal of the left molar area of the patient's teeth and places it on the microscopic slide. The chair-side assistant places 1 drop of distilled water on the plaque, positions the coverglass, and places it under the microscope.

6. Plaque is placed on a white tile and the D-K Caries Activity test is conducted.

A highly successful procedure is to demonstrate to the patient the characteristics of plaque. He is able to see that it is tooth color in appearance, sticky to remove, and it responds to color change when an acid indicator and sugar are added (D-K Caries Activity test). This demonstration will end with seeing the living bacteria under the microscope following the flossing procedure. It precedes the audiovisual presentation.

FIG. 7-10. The plaque in-
dex is scored from 0 to 3 from
left to right on the individual
teeth illustrated. The overall
appraisal of the dentition is
considered, in this text, to be
a plaque index of 2.

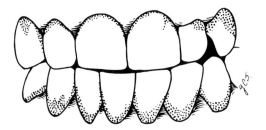

7. The dentist places Borofax on the lips of the patient.
8. Using the disclosant the patient discloses the plaque.
9. The chair-side assistant has the patient rinse his mouth well with water.
10. The chair-side assistant gives the patient the hand mirror, and the dentist points out to the patient the areas of plaque and

the other conditions relating to his disease. The areas without plaque are bright and shiny, and those with a bacterial coating are impregnated with coloring.

The decay process is brought to the patient's attention by scraping plaque from the tooth surface and then noting the whitish areas of decalcification found immediately under

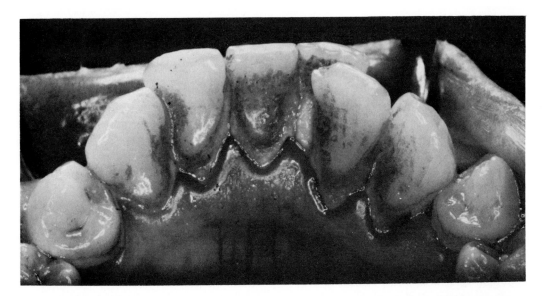

FIG. 7-11. The use of a disclosant to determine the plaque index. Without disclosing the plaque it could be considered as an oral hygiene evaluation. A calculus index is of assistance, and a numerical rating is given on the basis of each practitioner's judgment. We would score this 3, or heavy calculus accumulation.

the gummy mass. This is especially true along the borders of the gum and its extensions between the teeth. The different stages of decay can be viewed, from surface decalcification to further penetration of acids changing the colors from yellow to deep brown.

11. The plaque index is noted for the assistant to chart (Figs. 7-10, 7-11). This is done without explanation; it is for record purposes only. It is pointed out that the reason the dental plaque cannot be readily seen is the similar color of the plaque and the tooth.

12. As the patient observes in the hand mirror, the dentist, using unwaxed dental floss, flosses the teeth of the entire mouth and discusses with the patient areas of bleeding and tenderness. He points out the unmanageable areas involving inadequate restorations and periodontal pockets. The chair-side assistant charts on the patient's Test Record the facts observed.

It is suggested that the entire mouth be flossed at this visit. This cleaning of the interproximal areas of the teeth by the dentist gives the patient a good start in disorganizing the bacteria on the tooth surfaces and beneath the gums. The patient can see the conditions that exist in his entire mouth, the bleeding that takes place, the tenderness or soreness that is present, and he is able to taste and smell the bacterial waste products that are dislodged from between his teeth. These may also be areas where the floss breaks on rough restorations or other areas that need special attention. The dentist can provide suggestions in caring for these areas.

A suggested technique (see also Chapter 5): Wrap the floss around the index fingers and use these for the manipulation so that the patient can view the technique. Begin at the lower anterior teeth and progress to the right. This area is the easiest to demonstrate the presence of gum disease and the method of flossing.

These points are made to the patient as the flossing proceeds:

a. The gums may be sore in 3 to 4 days because the bacteria will be stirred up and the puffy gums will react to the change that is taking place, but continue flossing. This condition will improve, and in 5 or 6 days the bleeding will stop.

b. Be sure to get the dental floss all the way down underneath the gum.

c. Wrap the floss around the teeth so it cleans the entire side of the tooth.

d. After you get on to this you will be able to floss the teeth while watching television.

e. As you proceed to floss the upper anterior teeth, be sure that the floss is carried up until you meet resistance.

The flossing continues with the patient observing until all areas are flossed. Bridges are reserved until last.

After the flossing is completed, the patient can feel the difference and is beginning to sense what a clean tooth feels like and what it means to properly disorganize the bacteria.

13. The patient rinses his mouth.

14. The doctor and the patient view the bacterial plaque under the microscope (Fig. 7-12)

It helps to make a believer when the bacteria are observed under the phase microscope. The gelatinous mass becomes an active, living, wiggling clump of creatures with many different types of bacteria busily moving around. It is the activity observed that is the motivating factor along with the great numbers that are present. It is not important for the patient to know the names of the bacteria, but what is important is the direct contact that he receives with the smallest visible denominator of dental disease. This may be the beginning of the realization that his disease is a concern and that it should be properly treated and controlled.

If interest is shown, the difference between the organized and the disorganized bacteria may be demonstrated. White blood cells, red blood cells, and epithelial cells can also be related to the mechanism of dental disease in this way.

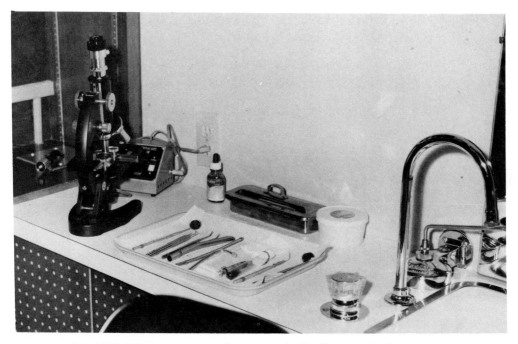

FIG. 7-12. The microscope and tray setup in the disease control operatory.

We do not live in a sterile world. We have to learn to live with bacteria. We have to learn to control them.

The observations that are made in the microscope should be noted and later recorded on the Test Record to provide an ongoing study and evaluation.

15. The chair-side assistant prepares the introduction filmstrip.
16. The dentist explains to the patient that he would like him to see this film, which is a summary of what has been said, after which the control therapist will help him. This allows the patient to rest and reflect on the new concepts that he has just been exposed to. It also helps to reinforce the information that he has received and serves to answer further questions of what is expected of him.
17. As soon as the filmstrip is completed the control therapist enters, introduces herself, turns off the projector, and invites the patient to leave the operatory and enter the control room.

Chapter 8 provides the step-by-step procedure for a control program from visit 1, part B through visit 8.

The disease control program is used to impart to the patient the knowledge of prevention and is the training ground to develop the skills necessary to preserve and maintain the oral tissue.

The Disease Control Program and Method of Delivery

Adequate time is required for each and every patient. Habits are not acquired in one day but are developed over a time. The patient is led through progressive steps of achievement so that he may learn the skills and effectively use the oral hygiene aids. These skills are not inherited but must be discovered and practiced to become a part of the patient's actions and behavior.

It is suggested that the professional staff not assume or take for granted the information to be presented. Chapter 5, Teaching Guide for Oral Hygiene, gives suggestions that should be experienced personally and critically evaluated. In regard to brushing the teeth, Dr. C. C. Bass deserves credit for providing that extra ingredient that so many times takes the ordinary and places it into the position of being better in performance and achievement. Techniques are continually being modified, and this is a sign of progress, but the starting point is a sound idea with a full application of the basic principles. The dentist must be sure that everyone on the dental staff thoroughly appreciates and practices each detail of the control program before it is presented to the patient.

In our society information is abundant but experience is lacking. One of the unique features of preventive dentistry and the control program is that it provides information and then follows through to provide a living experience. It is the achievement of short-range goals that motivates the patient to continue on a course that will ultimately lead to the long-range goal of not having dental decay and gum disease and keeping the teeth for a lifetime. It is the responsibility of the dental personnel to see that the patient arrives at the point in time when he realizes the advantages and is eager to accept and incorporate what is being taught into his own behavior.

As interest is aroused and questions develop, answers can be provided. If the solutions and data are relative to the patient's own thinking, more information will be readily accepted and tolerated by him. If what is being discussed is out of his realm of concern or his need to know, much more effort is required for acceptance and action.

The control program provides a check list to follow, and it is through such a framework of preventive information that the dental personnel can systematically and efficiently relate to the patient. It is carried out with empathy, firmness, expertise, and confidence in the techniques being presented.

DISEASE CONTROL
Visit 1, Part B

This visit is primarily a get-acquainted hour. The techniques and procedures are secondary. As the control therapist discusses the control program, confirms the patient's appointments, gives instruction on the dietary forms, explains his home supplies, and reviews once again the value of the disclosing tablet and the concepts of periodontal disease, she is getting to know the patient. The control therapist by her actions informs the patient that throughout the future sessions he will be held in high regard and that he can feel safe and secure in the knowledge that his self-respect will at all times be protected. It is this atmosphere of helpfulness that enables him to change habits and establish new ones that are conducive to maintaining oral health.

Time allowed for appointment: 60 minutes for the adult and 30 minutes for the child

Place: The control room

Persons involved: The patient and the control therapist

Goals:

1. To become acquainted with the patient.
2. To acquaint the patient with the disease control program.
3. To provide and discuss the significance of using proper oral hygiene supplies.
4. To acquaint the patient with the sulcular brushing techniques.

Equipment and supplies:

Items on the counter space for the patient to take home:

Appointment card (Fig. 3-11)

Pamphlet *Research Explores Plaque* (Fig. 5-50)

Nutritional evaluation questionnaire —Dietronics (Figs. 6-10, 6-11)

5-Day Food Diary (Fig. 6-9)

Prescription for home supplies and the supplies (Fig. 5-51)

Toothbrush, toothpaste, unwaxed dental floss, sixteen disclosing tablets, plastic dental mirror

Personal Oral Hygiene Instruction Sheet (Figs. 5-52, 5-53)

Instruction for home care, week 1 (Fig. 5-54)

Plastic bag for supplies

Visual aids on the counter top:

Models of the teeth and demonstration toothbrush

Picture of Procter and Gamble's Tablet Test

Picture showing the progression of periodontal disease (Fig. 4-4)

Supplies at the sink counter space:

Toothbrush with name tag

Toothpaste

Dental mouth mirror

Two flashlights; one regular type, one with a Floxite Mirror

Plastic disposable drinking cup

2 hand towels

Patient's chest towel and neck clip

Note: In order to remember the order of presentation, arrange the material in sequence of its use, the appointment card (with the appointments written in) on top and continuing with the instructions for home care week 1 on the bottom. The order and material to be included can be written on 3-by-5-inch cards and placed in an inconspicuous place where the control therapist can refer to them. If some information is forgotten it can be included at the following visit.

Procedure:

1. The control therapist greets the patient.
2. The five appointments made by the receptionist are confirmed. Appointments 6, 7, and 8 are explained. This discussion shows concern for the patient's time; it allows the two persons to adjust to each other, and it personally relates the appointments to the control therapist. The rapport that is established helps to prevent broken or canceled appointments.
3. Review the pamphlet *Research Explores Plaque* with the patient. Thumb through the pages and discuss the material and at which appointment the subjects will be presented.
4. Introduce the patient to and instruct him on how to complete the nutritional evaluation questionnaire. It is to be returned on visit 2.
5. Introduce the patient to and instruct him on how to complete the 5-Day Food Diary.

   Five days must elapse between visit 1 and visit 5. Include a Saturday, Sunday, or a holiday because food habits vary on these days. Keep instructions simple. Recall the food eaten by the patient for the past 24 hours and record. Stress that he should continue eating the same foods that he is accustomed to eating and not to change his food selection.

The Dietronics form is reviewed with the patient before the discussion of the 5-Day Food Diary because it is the simplest and requires the least amount of time to complete. The 5-Day Food Diary is time consuming and somewhat complicated. If the 5-Day Food Diary is presented first, the patient, while wondering how he will ever write down everything he eats, is not receptive to further instructions of another form. If the adult male remarks that he does not have time to complete either form, suggest that his wife do it. He will hasten to remark that he guesses he can do it, and he will.

6. Using the prescription form for home supplies, discuss with the patient the supplies that he is to take home.
   a. The toothbrush
      Ask the patient to discard the toothbrush he has been using. If he has just purchased a new toothbrush (this happens frequently), reassure him that the toothbrush that he receives is a good toothbrush and that he will like it. He will receive three brushes during the control program —one to take home, the second to be used by him at each visit at the office (this is taken home on the 1-month visit), and the third brush is given to the patient on the 2-month visit.
   b. The dental floss
      Show the patient the three types of dental floss, thin unwaxed, heavy unwaxed, and waxed.
   c. The disclosing tablets
      These are used as a teaching aid to learn the technique, and thereafter they serve as a check. Give sixteen tablets to each patient. It seems fairly consistent that most families share the disclosant with other mem-

bers during the first week. If an insufficient number is given on the first visit, the patient will ask for more to complete his 2-week experience.
   d. Miscellaneous supplies not appearing on the prescription form
      Toothpaste: A fluoride paste should be used because fluoride contributes to the resistance of the tooth to decay. Further discussion will be held on visit 4.
      Mouth mirror: It is used to view the inside of the mouth. Some patients will be able to use it; others will not, depending upon their eyesight.
      Floss threaders: These are given to patients who have bridges or splinted teeth. The patient will be assisted with its use in visit 2.
   All supplies are put into a plastic bag and placed in a convenient place for the patient to take home.

7. Discuss with the patient the visual aid Tablet Test. The first in the series, Before Tablet Test, is usually what the teeth look like when first seen by the dental staff. Indicate that everyone's teeth are being referred to and not specifically this patient's teeth. The patient's self-respect must be preserved or he will be unable to receive the information being offered.

In the second of the series, After Tablet Test, point out the amount of bacteria that accumulates in about 24 hours (upper anterior teeth) and the amount of bacteria that accumulates in several days (upper back teeth). Indicate that this is what the teeth look like when they feel furry to the tongue, and, if appropriate, indicate that this is the area that most children often miss when brushing their teeth because the lip is strong and the hand is weak. Unless an effort is made on the part of the child only the area near the biting surface is cleaned.

In discussing the final picture in this

series, After Brushing Properly, stress the fact that the teeth glisten not because of the use of the pink tablet but because the bacteria have been removed, and that the patient's teeth will shine too in about 5 to 6 days, even teeth that have not been cleaned by the dentist or hygienist and that are stained from coffee and tea. This statement gives the patient hope and provides a short-range goal for him to achieve.

Patients may ask if it was not the pink tablet that made the teeth shine. This may be because glistening teeth have not been within their experience. Most teeth will shine before the 5 days, but this allows a margin of safety and provides an opportunity to accomplish the goal early as well as for the patient to receive the much needed praise from the control therapist.

8. Discuss the meaning of the visual aid, progression of periodontal disease (Fig. 4-4).

The first picture in the series shows the inflammation of the gums caused by the waste products of the bacteria that are attached to the tooth or filling. The second shows pocket formation and beginning bone loss. The third picture illustrates the severe bone loss of the late stages with possible loss of the tooth. Point out to the patient the bacterial mass that he will be disorganizing and removing every day with the dental floss and the toothbrush bristle. As the bacteria grow back their waste products will flow out into the mouth instead of being held tight against the tooth as is the case when the bacteria have been left undisturbed in an organized mass. The bone will not come back but the infection leaves the gums and the gum will clamp onto the tooth, making a loose tooth tighter. This improvement occurs within approximately 10 days. Have the patient understand that the greater the bone loss, the greater the mobility, and that there is a point at which there may be insufficient bone to support the tooth.

Pyorrhea is a word most adults know but do not understand. Children recognize the condition as being different and are eager to know what it is and why it is dreaded by so many relatives. The patient appreciates this story because now he knows what pyorrhea is. Using an indirect approach, stress to the patient the importance of flossing each day.

It is necessary to reassure a patient who already has severe periodontal disease. This can be done by telling him that we cannot worry about what has gone on in the past; we are concerned with now and the future, and we will help him to learn how to control his disease. This assurance is important to relieve the patient of unnecessary guilt feelings.

9. Review and discuss with the patient the Personal Oral Hygiene Instruction Sheet.
   a. Review *To Show Bacterial Colonies* and *Inspection* of the mouth.
   b. Return to *Brushing* and *Flossing* after completing the review of the entire instruction sheet. This is followed by a demonstration of the brushing technique on the models and a return demonstration by the patient in his own mouth.
   c. *Rinsing:* Tell the patient that if he has a water spray, it would be used at this time.
   d. *Reinspection:* Remove any remaining areas of bacterial plaque.
   e. *General information:* The best time to clean the teeth is at bedtime. There is less saliva in the mouth during the night hours, and saliva serves to flush and rinse the mouth. Bacteria do not live well in saliva but do grow well in warm, dark, moist areas that are left undisturbed.

   If it is more convenient to clean the teeth during the daytime, this is permissible. Mothers of young children may wish to clean their teeth during the day before the tiring bedtime hours. It can be suggested that the patient clean his teeth before going out in the evening rather than after coming home late. The patient will many times be too tired to do a good cleaning, if he does it at all, and this skipping can be devastating to habit formation. Cleaning the teeth before a social engagement so they will look their best can be suggested as a further incentive.

State that the gums may be tender and sore during the first 2 weeks of this program because the infection that is present may be stirred up.

f. *The measure of success:* Inform the patient that it is necessary to clean the teeth once in 24 hours because it takes that long for the bacteria to grow back and organize once they have been removed.

10. Review the home care for weeks 1, 2, and 3, and instruct the patient on week 1.

11. Flossing: Ask the patient if he has ever used dental floss. This informs how difficult the task will be at visit 2 and how much time will be needed.

Instruct the patient not to floss again today because the dentist has already flossed his entire mouth. The exception is children. Children need to practice, and the newly awakened enthusiasm should not be stifled.

Assure the patient that he will be assisted on the next visit. If for some unavoidable reason he is not to be seen the following day, review the flossing technique, and at the time of brushing have him demonstrate in his own mouth by flossing several teeth on the upper and the lower arch. Tell him to do the best he can but not to be concerned if it is difficult and that he will have help at his next visit.

12. Using the demonstration tooth models, review the old toothbrushing technique (up on the lower and down on the upper, brushing as they grow). This has been an awkward and a difficult procedure. The hand must rotate up and outward on the lower and inward on the upper arch. Consequently, many people throughout their lifetime have not even attempted it. More important is that the bacteria live in the area where the tooth meets the gums (sulcus), and with the old method the area is swept over and the bacteria left undisturbed. The patient has to understand what is wrong with his old way before he will accept a new method.

Demonstrate the sulcular brushing technique. Do not forget to brush the tongue!

13. Invite the patient to take his place at the sink and, using the new method, remove the "pink" from his teeth.

Brushing the teeth in the presence of another person can be very difficult and embarrassing for some patients. If a patient is to learn the technique properly, he must brush them here; it is at this first visit that the patient meets and subsequently adjusts to this difficult situation. As the control therapist observes the patient, she should be reserved and allow him ample room. If the patient is sitting, she should be sitting so that they are on the same level.

14. Have the patient wash his hands if he desires.

15. Place the chest towel on the patient.

16. Indicate to the patient the toothbrush and paste that he will be using during his visits. Have the patient wet the toothbrush and add a small amount of toothpaste.

17. Demonstrate the brushing technique in the patient's mouth in the lower left molar area and in the lower lingual anterior area.

18. Have the patient brush all his teeth using the new brushing technique. Remind him to brush his tongue.

19. Have the patient rinse his mouth. Assure him that after the technique has been perfected he will be able to floss

and brush his teeth in less than 5 minutes.

20. The control therapist washes her hands.
21. The patient, using a flashlight with a Floxite mirror, and the control therapist, using a second flashlight and a dental mouth mirror, together examine the teeth for pink. All areas of plaque may not have been removed. Large areas of plaque, such as might be found on the lingual of the lower back molars, may be further brushed for removal; otherwise, what remains can be removed at the next appointment.

    The brushing of the teeth on this visit should be to acquaint the patient with the technique. In all probability this technique is strange and difficult and the patient is tired.
22. Ask the patient a specific question, "How do your teeth feel?" He will feel his teeth with his tongue and say, "Very good." This is important because he is beginning to note what his teeth really feel like.

    An important motivational factor in the control program is this feel and noting the change from a dirty mouth to a clean mouth. The patient cannot appreciate this until he notices the difference in feel, taste, and smell.
23. The patient may wash his hands again if he desires.
24. The control therapist washes her hands.
25. Remove the chest towel from the patient.
26. Ask the patient not to clean his teeth before he comes in for visit 2 because he will be cleaning them at this appointment. Suggest that he may brush the food off in the evening before bed but he should not floss or do the sulcular brushing. It is well if 24 hours elapse before brushing again to allow recovery of the gingival tissue, and this will help to make the mouth less tender.

    Some patients, enthusiastic with their new tools, will repeat the technique. This the control therapist has no control over; however, it should be stressed that it takes 24 hours for the bacteria to grow back in sufficient numbers and that it really is not necessary. The important thing is that the patient is starting a habit change to a once-a-day thorough cleaning. At visit 2 the control therapist will want the patient to see and feel how clean the teeth are or how "dirty" they get in 24 hours. If he has brushed them several times since his last visit, he will have lost this phase of awareness.

27. Confirm the appointment for visit 2. State that the visit the following day will be shorter, approximately 45 minutes. By informing the patient of the length of the appointment, he is better able to plan his time. Inform him that assistance will be given in the use of floss, and the correct use of the toothpick will be discussed.

    A preview of the next appointment gives him something to think about and to look forward to. Patients arrive on time for appointments, even early, eager with anticipation. *Caution:* Do not tell the patient what will be done on the following visit if there is a possibility that it will not be accomplished.

    The patient has been under stress and has perhaps exerted great emotional energy during this appointment, and as he leaves, the control therapist should thank him, in her actions, for what he has accomplished. The patient is handed his supplies and escorted to the reception room.

    The control therapist receives satisfaction for the tremendous effort she gave to make this visit a success through the grateful thank-you as the patient bids her good-bye and says he will see her tomorrow.

28. Charting
    a. Complete the patient's chart and write recommendations for the following visit.
    b. Make entries in the specific record books that the office is keeping, for example, a notebook listing all new

DISEASE CONTROL CHECK LIST

Name _____

Chart # _____ Age _____

Grade of school _____

Diagnosis _____

Disease Control Visit # 1, Date _____

Phase Microscope used _____

Film, "Secrets of the Little World" _____

Dietronics Questionnaire _____

Five Day Food Diary _____

Home supplies _____

Oral Hygiene Instruction _____

Floss _____ Brush _____

Other _____

Records: Patient's Log, Nutritional Log, KEY

Visit # 2, Date _____

Return Dietronics Questionnaire _____

Oral Hygiene Instruction _____

Floss _____ Floss threader _____

Stain _____ Brush _____

Proxabrush _____ Other _____

Patient smokes _____ Stain remover _____

Condition of gums _____

Demonstration of Perio-Aid _____

Educational pamphlet _____

Other _____

Visit # 3, Date _____

Saliva Tests _____

Oral Hygiene Instruction _____

Floss _____ Floss threader _____

Perio-Aid _____ Stain _____

Brush _____ Proxabrush _____

Water Spray _____

Other _____

Condition of gums _____

Demonstration of water sprays _____

Patient has a water spray _____

Type _____

Water Spray recommended _____

Other _____

FIG. 8-1. The Disease Control Check List. Each part is accompanied by a tooth chart like those in Figure 8-2.

patients; a notebook listing the nutritional evaluation; an address list for office publications such as *The Key* or Christmas cards.

The Disease Control Check List (Figs. 8-1 to 8-3) facilitates the conducting of the procedures. In using the tooth chart section of this form, the pocket areas are marked in green, the areas of bleeding resulting from flossing and brushing are marked in red, and the areas of plaque remaining after cleaning are marked in blue.

If the patient is to be assisted in areas of poor technique, they must first be identified. It is impossible to remember each patient's peculiarities so for the purpose of record it is charted. It also becomes a part of his permanent legal record.

Recommendations to be used on the continuing visits are made on the Personal Observation Record (Fig. 8-4).

DISEASE CONTROL
Visit 2

Time allowed for appointment: 45 minutes

Place: The control room

Persons involved: The patient and the control therapist

Short-range goals:

1. To assist the patient with the flossing technique.
2. To assist in establishing a systematic method in brushing the teeth.
3. To demonstrate how to remove excessive stains.
4. To demonstrate how and when to use a toothpick properly.
5. To become better acquainted with the patient.

Throughout this visit the control therapist should be mindful of the friendship that is being established. She must be conscious of the information that is required to personalize this program and the methods by which she intends to obtain it. This seems to be best obtained through informal conversation.

Visit # 4, Date _____
Rx Home Care Week # 2 _____
Oral Hygiene Instruction _____
Floss _____ Floss threader _____
Perio-Aid _____ Brush _____
Proxabrush _____ Stain _____
Water Spray _____ Other _____
Condition of gums _____
Pamphlet "What You Need to Know. ." _____
Discussion of General Dentistry _____
Discussion of patient's oral conditions _____
Other _____

Visit # 5, Date _____
Return Food Diary, Late _____
Oral Glucose Clearance Test _____
Discussion of "Preventive Measures. ." _____
Discussion of Snyder Test and results _____
Discussion of "What Should I Eat?" _____
Discussion of "Hidden Sugars" _____
Snack List developed _____
"Snack Suggestions" given to patient _____
Rx Home Care Week # 2 _____
Oral Hygiene Instructions _____
Floss _____ Floss threader _____
Perio-Aid _____ Brush _____
Proxabrush _____ Stain _____
Water Spray _____ Other _____
Condition of gums _____
Other _____

Visit # 6, Date _____
Program presented to parent _____
Film, "Judy's. . Notebook"-child - _____
Film, "Vitamins and You"-Adol. - _____
Discussion RDA and related material _____
Discussion of Nutritional Evaluation _____
"Daily Check-List of Nutrients"-adult _____
"Dietary Evaluation" - all patients - _____
"A Guide to Good Eating" - all patients - _____
"Your Food-Chance or Choice"-Adol.- _____
Food Models - all except adults- _____
Fact sheets- adults- _____

Rx Home Care Week # 3 _____
Oral Hygiene Instruction _____
Floss _____ Floss threader _____
Perio-Aid _____ Brush _____
Proxabrush _____ Stain-Plak-Lite _____
Water Spray _____ Other _____
Condition of gums _____

Bleeding-red Plaque-blue Perio pocket-green

FIG. 8-2. The Disease Control Check List (*Continued*).

Visit # 7, Date _____
Snyder Test # 2 _____
Fifteen Minute Caries Test _____
Oral Hygiene Instruction _____
Floss _____ Floss threader _____
Frequency _____
Perio-Aid _____ Frequency _____
Stain-two color dye _____
_____ Frequency _____
Brush _____ Frequency _____
Proxabrush _____ Frequency _____
Water Spray _____ Frequency _____
Other _____
Condition of gums _____
Discussion of foods _____
Supplements being taken _____
Booklet "Boy and His Physique" - Adol. _____
Booklet "Girl and Her Figure" - Adol. _____
Other _____
Home supplies _____
Response to Disease Control
    Good   Fair   Poor

Visit # 8, Date _____
Snyder Test # 3 _____
Oral Hygiene Instruction _____
Floss _____ Floss threader _____
Frequency _____
Perio-Aid _____ Frequency _____
Stain-two color dye _____
_____ Frequency _____
Brush _____ Frequency _____
Proxabrush _____ Frequency _____
Water Spray _____ Frequency _____
Other _____
Condition of gums _____
Discussion of foods _____
Home supplies _____
Recall _____
Other _____

FIG. 8-3. The Disease Control Check List (*Continued*). (Each part requires an accompanying tooth chart as in Figure 8-2).

Long-range goal:
To have the patient associate flossing with the brushing of the teeth.
Equipment:
Counter space:
  Models of teeth with demonstration brush
  Perio-Aid with toothpicks
  Ajax and Q-tips

Pamphlet *A New Plan to Keep Your Teeth for a Lifetime* (see Fig. 5-58) and *The Prevention Key* (see Fig. 3-21)
Patient's chart
Sink counter space:
  Two hand towels
  The patient's chest towel and neck clip
  Patient's toothbrush and Proxabrush, Floss holder, and Floss threader as needed
  Patient's toothpaste
  Diagnostic models of the patient's teeth
  Mouth mirror
  Patient's drinking cup
  Disclosing tablet
  Vaseline on 2-by-2-inch gauze
  Dental floss
  Flashlights
Procedure:
1. The control therapist greets the patient. The patient returns the nutritional evaluation questionnaire.
2. Have the patient wash his hands.
3. Have the patient be seated.
4. Using the demonstration models of the teeth, demonstrate the proper flossing technique.

    Mothers use the floss holder in flossing the teeth of children between 2 and 5 years of age. The holder allows the mother to clean swiftly and effectively in a mouth that is small; it has to be done quickly because a child is impatient. Children 5 to 7 years may use a floss holder. Children from the third grade and older learn to finger the floss. Adults, unless physically handicapped, are not given a holder until they prove that they cannot floss without it.

5. Have the patient floss all his teeth. Floss threaders are used to clean under bridges and splinted teeth.

    A patient learns where "his teeth are" and how to manipulate the floss without interference from the control therapist. The patient believes he can do it, he has a strong desire to do it, and it is essential that he do it even if it is extremely sloppy.

    Delay judgment and evaluation of the patient's ability to handle floss for several days. The improvements that are made are unbelievable.

All patients may not perfect the technique within the 2 weeks of the control program. It is a skill that is worked at and improved each time it is done, and this is for the lifetime of the tooth.

6. Have the patient rinse his mouth.
7. Place the chest towel on the patient.
8. Have the patient put Vaseline on his lips and fingers to prevent staining from the disclosant.
9. The patient stains his teeth with the disclosant and rinses his mouth. Dentures and appliances are left in the mouth for staining.
10. The control therapist washes her hands.
11. Have the patient remove appliances.
12. The control therapist and the patient, each using flashlights and mirror, together inspect the teeth and discuss what they see. Ascertain from the patient the last time his teeth were brushed. Point out the areas of greatest stain, giving spe-

PERSONAL OBSERVATION RECORD

Name _____

Date	Visit # 1
Observations	
Recommendations	
Date	Visit # 2
Observations	
Recommendations	
Date	Visit # 3
Observations	
Recommendations	
Date	Visit # 4
Observations	
Recommendations	
Date	Visit # 5
Observations	
Recommendations	
Date	Visit # 6
Observations	
Recommendations	
Date	Visit # 7
Observations	
Recommendations	

Comments:

FIG. 8-4. Personal Observation Record (adapted from PBP).

cial attention to the gum line of the teeth on both the tongue and cheek side. Have the patient compare the amount of stain on the teeth today with the amount disclosed on visit 1. Ask the patient if his teeth feel dirty. His answer in all probability will be no.

The patient is beginning to realize that his teeth do not really get very dirty in 24 hours and that, in fact, it does take time for these living bacteria to grow. He further realizes the toothbrushing he had been doing was not really very good. It is important that the patient decide this for himself, he is not being told, nor is he being threatened into learning this new cleaning procedure. He is being respected as an intelligent individual who has the ability and the capacity to motivate himself to use the techniques.

This observation period is concluded by evaluating the amount of bacteria that will accumulate in a given period. Inform the patient that this is his plaque pattern, that it is peculiar to him, and it will always remain basically the same. That is why we can learn how to remove it by the use of disclosants and carry this knowledge over into daily practice.

13. Demonstrate on the patient's diagnostic models the sulcular brushing technique.

Patients desire to do the techniques properly, but they may not remember the details. To prevent embarrassment and provide reinforcement, the flossing and brushing techniques are demonstrated at each visit.

Suggest that the gum brush not be used to clean removable appliances. To effectively clean an appliance, household cleansers and a hard-bristle toothbrush are used. The Proxabrush is used in areas of periodontal involvement.

14. Have the patient brush all of his teeth. Carefully suggest changes in his technique in areas needing improvement. This can be done by directing his movement in his mouth or by showing him on his own diagnostic models.

Have the patient clean the appliances and remind him to brush his tongue. Some patients will forget to clean the tongue until they have established the systematic method of brushing. Adults may be embarrassed by having someone watch them brush their tongue. The control therapist can become busy to provide the privacy necessary for the patient.

15. Show the patient how to remove stains from the teeth. A small amount of household cleanser such as Ajax is placed on a moistened Q-tip. Caution the patient not to use this as toothpaste or toothpowder to clean the entire dentition because it is very abrasive. Its use is to be very limited. If there is bleeding of the gums, this demonstration is delayed until all bleeding has ceased.

16. Have the patient rinse his mouth well with a cup of warm water to remove the material he has loosened with the floss and the toothbrush. If there has been a great deal of bleeding or the gums are tender, have him use a rinse of ½ teaspoon salt to 1 cup of warm water. Suggest that he use this at home also.

The saline solution is soothing and healing, but, more important, it is something special that has been done by him. By carrying out this procedure at home, the patient is doing something familiar that will help himself. It must be remembered that at this point in the control program the patient does not believe 100 per cent that the "piece of string" and the brush will stop the bleeding and make the gums stop hurting. This fact has not been proven to him; it has only been told to him.

17. The control therapist washes her hands.

18. The patient and the control therapist together inspect the teeth for the remaining bacterial mass. Have the patient feel his teeth with his tongue.

The teeth will feel smooth and clean; the mouth will tingle. The patient is beginning to learn what clean teeth feel like, and this awareness is essential for him in obtaining the motivation that will enable him to change his habits.

19. Have the patient wash his hands if he desires. The control therapist washes her hands.
20. Remove the chest towel from the patient.
21. Show the patient how to use the toothpick correctly. A child patient should be taught this too.

    The toothpick can cause damage if it is jabbed into the tissue. Patients should be aware of this. The toothpick is placed into the Perio-Aid or Proxabrush handle for easier use.

    The toothpick's primary use is in areas of pocket formation and in areas of bleeding that have not been controlled by the use of the floss and the toothbrush within 4 or 5 days into the program.

    Using his models, show the patient how to clean under tipped teeth, along the linguals of the back molars, and other difficult cleaning areas. The toothpick can also be used to clean the lingual surfaces of children's teeth. The cleaning in pocket formations is shown only if it is specific for that mouth. It is stressed that dental floss is used to remove any food that is lodged between the teeth while eating and that the toothpick is used to remove bacterial plaque.
22. Provide specific home instructions as needed.

    Ask the patient *not to floss until the next day* unless the flossing was extremely difficult and inadequate, in which case suggest he practice that evening. This is especially true with children.

    If several days will elapse before visit 3, write specific instructions on the dentist's prescription form (see Fig. 5-57).
23. Provide the patient with copies and an explanation of *The Prevention Key* and *A New Plan to Keep Your Teeth for a Lifetime.*
24. Inform the patient that the next appointment will be approximately 1 hour, and it will include a demonstration of water sprays.

25. Dismiss the patient by confirming his next appointment. Walk with him to the reception room.
26. Charting
    a. Indicate areas of plaque (after cleaning), bleeding, and tenderness on Disease Control Check List.
    b. Make recommendations for visit 3 on Personal Observation Record.

    Give the nutritional evaluation questionnaire to the receptionist for mailing.

DISEASE CONTROL
Visit 3

Time allowed for appointment: approximately 60 minutes
Place: The control room
Persons involved: The patient, the control therapist, and auxiliary
Goals:
1. To stress that the floss must be carried under the margins of the gingival tissue, wrapped around the tooth, and kept tight against the tooth as it is scraped.
2. To assist the patient in perfecting sulcular cleaning.
3. To demonstrate the various types of water sprays and discuss their use and value.
Equipment:
Counter space:
  2 graduated cylinders for saliva testing
  Models of teeth with demonstration toothbrush
  Water sprays for demonstration
  Patient's chart with Test Record (Fig. 4-6)
Sink counter space:
  Two hand towels
  The patient's chest towel and neck clip
  Patient's toothbrush and Proxabrush, Floss threader, Floss holder and Perio-Aid as needed
  Patient's toothpaste
  Diagnostic models of the patient's teeth
  Mouth mirror
  Patient's drinking cup
  Disclosing tablet
  Vaseline on 2-by-2-inch gauze
  Dental floss
  Flashlights

Procedure:

1. The control therapist greets the patient.
2. Have the patient wash his hands.
3. Have the patient be seated.
4. Place the chest towel on the patient.
5. Have the patient collect unstimulated saliva in a graduated cylinder for 5 minutes. Record the amount on the Test Record.
6. Have the patient chew paraffin and collect the stimulated saliva in a graduated cylinder for 5 minutes. Record the amount on the Test Record. A total of 10 ml. is needed for saliva testing—extend the time if necessary to collect this amount.

   The saliva is taken immediately upon collection to the test center. Testing is done by another staff member. Inform the patient that the tests are being conducted to assist in determining the factors involved in his disease and to help determine the course to follow in controlling it. The test results are given to him in visits 5 and 6.
7. Demonstrate the flossing technique on the demonstration models.
8. Have the patient floss his teeth using floss threader and holder as needed.

   The bleeding will be greatly reduced. Mention should be made of this fact, and it should be stated again that this bleeding is due to the action of the bacterial waste products on the gums. The control therapist should not feel discouraged when, even in view of previous conversations, the patient says, "My gums bled last night because I cut them with the floss." This comment should be followed immediately by a statement of the actual cause of bleeding gums. The handling of the floss has become less cumbersome and the cleaning more effective.
9. Have the patient use the Perio-Aid (toothpick) as needed.
10. Have the patient rinse his mouth.
11. Have the patient put Vaseline on his lips and fingers to prevent staining from the disclosant.
12. Have the patient stain his teeth with the disclosant with appliances inserted. Have him rinse his mouth.
13. The control therapist washes her hands.
14. Have patient remove appliances.
15. The patient and the control therapist discuss and inspect the teeth and the appliances for plaque.
16. Demonstrate on the patient's diagnostic models the sulcular technique. Stress that the bristles are not to be "dragged" across the gum tissue, but rather they are placed, vibrated, picked up, and then replaced. Determine if there are any areas of tenderness.

    Tenderness of the gums can be experienced either at the onset of the program or in 7 to 10 days into the program. If tenderness is present during the beginning visits, it is important that the patient have the daily supportive attention of the control therapist. If the patient is left to floss and brush his teeth alone, he will not do it because of this tenderness.
17. Have the patient brush all his teeth and tongue. The Proxabrush is used as needed.

    The patient must floss and brush all the teeth, even areas of tenderness. Many times this "hurt" that is expressed by the patient will feel good during the cleaning procedure. Inform the patient that this tenderness is due to the infection that has been stirred up.
18. Have the patient rinse his mouth, using warm salt water if the gums are tender.
19. The control therapist washes her hands.
20. The patient and the control therapist again inspect the teeth and the appliances for plaque.
21. Both the patient and the control therapist wash their hands.
22. Remove the chest towel from the patient.
23. Show water irrigators to the patient. Discuss and demonstrate them so he understands their purpose, and becomes knowledgeable as to their use. Explain that the irrigation removes the bacterial waste products, toxins, and material

loosened by the flossing and brushing. This irrigation of the sulcular area around the teeth also washes away the serum that has been discharged by the subgingival tissue that feeds the bacteria.

Our policy is to encourage all patients in the use of water irrigation. It is recommended for all patients with periodontal involvement.

Demonstrate the desired water pressure as it flows from the tip of the irrigator. It is desirable not to force the bacteria back into the gingival tissues or into the bloodstream. The force should be gentle yet strong enough to remove the waste materials.

The use of water sprays is delayed until all bleeding is controlled.

24. Give home instructions as needed.
25. Confirm the appointment for visit 4. Time required will be 45 minutes. The topics to be discussed are the value and use of fluorides, x-rays, and dental disease as it concerns the patient.
26. Dismiss the patient.
27. Charting
    a. Indicate areas of plaque (after cleaning), bleeding, and tenderness on Disease Control Check List.
    b. Make recommendations for visit 4 on Personal Observation Record.

DISEASE CONTROL
Visit 4

Time allowed for appointment: 45 minutes
Place: The control room
Persons involved: The patient and the control therapist
Short-range goals:
1. To closely observe the flossing technique and correct as necessary.
2. To closely observe the brushing technique and correct as necessary.
3. To obtain a history of the patient's daily activities.
4. To instill appreciation and understanding of the oral hygiene technique through use of basic dental science.
5. To encourage patient motivation by personalizing the program through the

use of the patient's x-rays, chart, and diagnostic models.
Long-range goals:
1. To have the patient realize the significance of oral disease.
2. To have the patient realize that it applies to him.
3. To have the patient understand that it is through his own efforts, not the dentist's that dental disease is controlled.
Equipment:
Counter space:
    Models of teeth with demonstration brush
    Visual aids: Structure of the tooth; progression of dental decay (see Fig. 4-1)
    Pamphlet *What You Need to Know and Do to Prevent Dental Caries (Tooth Decay) and Periodontal Disease (Pyorrhea)* (see Fig. 5-59)
    Prescription for home care week 2 (see Fig. 5-55)
    Patient's chart and Nutritional Record (see Fig. 6-25)
Sink counter space:
    Two hand towels
    The patient's chest towel and neck clip
    Patient's toothbrush and Proxabrush, Floss threader, Floss holder, Perio-Aid and water irrigator as needed
    Patient's toothpaste
    Diagnostic models of the patient's teeth
    Mouth mirror
    Patient's drinking cup
    Disclosing tablet
    Vaseline on 2-by-2-inch gauze
    Dental floss
    Flashlights
Procedure:
1. The control therapist greets the patient.
2. Have the patient wash his hands.
3. Have the patient be seated.
4. Review with the patient the instructions for home care week 2 (these procedures assist him in establishing the habit of daily flossing and brushing of his teeth):
    Clean the teeth at the same time each day. This is helpful but not essential. The individual should establish the time that is best for him.
    Floss first then brush. This helps to

insure that the flossing is accomplished each day. Flossing can be done any time during the 24 hours that it is convenient, but it must be done.

Always start in the same place and follow a set pattern. This trains the hand so that it is not necessary to remember what has been done and what remains to be finished.

5. Demonstrate the flossing technique on the demonstration models. *Stress* carrying the floss deep, wrapping it around the tooth, and keeping it tight on the tooth as it is scraped.
6. Have the patient floss all his teeth using floss, holder, and threader as needed. Observe the technique closely and correct as necessary.
7. Have the patient use the Perio-Aid as needed.
8. Have the patient rinse his mouth.
9. Place the chest towel on the patient.
10. Demonstrate the toothbrushing technique on the patient's diagnostic models. Have children demonstrate the technique on the models before brushing their teeth. Correct the technique as needed.
11. Have the patient brush all his teeth, using the Proxabrush as needed. Clean the appliances.
12. Comment on the shiny appearance of the teeth. The patient will usually respond, "Yes, my husband noticed or my mother has made mention of it." An exception to this may be a negative reply by a spouse who is edentulous. It can be explained to the patient that many times a person who lacks teeth feels left out and cannot appreciate what another person is accomplishing through this program. It could be further explained that an edentulous patient can benefit through a control program that has been modified to meet his needs.
13. Discuss with the patient the general feel of his teeth and mouth as compared to 1 week ago. Some patients will think a moment and reply in the affirmative;

others, it will seem, are just waiting to be asked and respond with much enthusiasm and fervor. For the patient to continue to floss daily, he must realize that it is his need to do so. It is for this reason that he acknowledges the changes that have occurred in his mouth during the first 3 to 4 days of the Control Program.

14. Have the patient put Vaseline on his lips and fingers to prevent staining from the disclosant.
15. Have the patient stain his teeth and appliances and rinse his mouth.
16. The control therapist washes her hands.
17. The patient and the control therapist inspect the teeth and appliances for plaque. Technique may be altered to meet the needs.
18. Have the patient brush the teeth and tongue to remove excessive color.
19. The control therapist washes her hands.
20. Have the patient use the water irrigator if recommended by the dentist.
21. Remove the chest towel from the patient.
22. Have the patient wash his hands if he desires.
23. Invite the patient to the area specified for discussion.

The patient is ready for this information because rapport has been established. The time involved in cleaning the teeth has been shortened, and there is now time for other things. The patient realizes he has teeth and where they are; some may be crooked and hard to clean. He sees the conditions that exist and is ready to learn what he can do to correct it. In addition to this, the control therapist will gain valuable insight into the patient's desires and attitudes toward dentistry. The patient will discuss with the control therapist topics that he will not discuss with the dentist.

Through this discussion the control therapist instills the reasons specific oral hygiene aids and techniques are necessary to control the disease in his mouth. It prepares him for the dental treatment to be done now and in the future.

24. Using the visual aid, review the anatomy of a normal tooth.
25. Discuss the value and use of fluorides.
26. Using the visual aid, discuss the progression of decay.
27. Discuss the value and the use of x-rays.
28. Discuss saliva and its relationship to decay.
29. Present and review with the patient the pamphlet *What You Need to Know to Prevent Dental Caries (Tooth Decay) and Periodontal Disease (Pyorrhea)*.

    By this visit the patient through his own experience can understand and appreciate its content. He can relate those experiences discussed in the pamphlet with himself, his family, and his friends.
30. Review with the patient the decay and periodontal disease that exists in his mouth. Show him on his diagnostic models how the cleaning procedures prevent the accumulation of the decay-producing bacteria. Discuss and answer questions concerning his treatment plan. If he is a parent or grandparent and is interested, discuss children's dentistry.
31. Complete Section I and II of the Nutritional Record. This information is used in preparation for visits 5 and 6.
32. Confirm the following appointment. Time required will be 1 hour. Remind the patient to return his 5-Day Food Diary. The discussion will concern the foods we eat that are also food for the bacteria.
33. Dismiss the patient.
34. Charting
    a. Indicate any areas of plaque (after cleaning), bleeding, and tenderness on Disease Control Check List.
    b. Make recommendations for next visit on Personal Observation Record.

DISEASE CONTROL
Visit 5

Time allowed for appointment: 60 minutes
Place: The control room
Persons involved: The patient and the control therapist
Short-range goals:
1. To learn the foods that feed the decay-producing bacteria.
2. To identify these foods in the diet.
3. To substitute these foods for ones containing more nutrients that will enhance health.
Long-range goal:
   To have the patient alter or change his food selections and those of his family so that they can live in harmony in this "sugar world."
Equipment:
Counter space:
   Models of teeth with demonstration toothbrush
   Visual aid: Chart, Tablet Test
   Take-home packet for the patient that includes the following:
      Prescription for home care week 2 if not given to patient on visit 4.
      Worksheet, Preventive Measures for Your Dental Health (Figs. 6-14, 6-15)
      5-Day Food Diary that has been returned by the patient
      List, Hidden Sugar: Carbohydrate Evaluation (Fig. 6-6)
      List, What Should I Eat? (Figs. 6-16, 6-17)
      List, Party Time Snacks (Fig. 6-19)
      Picture, Your Snacks: Chance or Choice? (Fig. 6-5)
      Appointment card for visit 6
   Patient's Snyder test
   Oral glucose clearance test — Tes-Tape, candy bar, timer
   Patient's chart with results of saliva viscosity, saliva flow, Snyder test, and acid-buffering capacity of saliva
Sink counter space:
   Two hand towels

The patient's chest towel and neck clip
Patient's toothbrush and Proxabrush, Floss threader, Floss holder, Perio-Aid and water irrigator as needed
Patient's toothpaste
Diagnostic models of the patient's teeth
Mouth mirror
Patient's drinking cup
Disclosing tablet
Vaseline on 2-by-2-inch gauze
Dental floss
Flashlights

Procedure:

1. The control therapist greets the patient. The 5-Day Food Diary is returned.

2. Explain to the patient that in order to conduct the oral glucose clearance test the cleaning of the teeth will be delayed until the close of the visit. This test is conducted on all patients except diabetics. It is used primarily as a motivational tool. It enables the patient to *visualize* the length of time the sugar stays in the mouth.

3. As the test is being conducted (approximately 30 minutes) discuss with the patient the relationship that exists between refined carbohydrates and decay.

4. Using the worksheet, Preventive Measures for Your Dental Health, discuss its content. This form is fan folded. Page 1: Name and date. Page 6: To keep my teeth for my lifetime
   Page 2: My dental concern:
   Review with the patient his primary concern. It may be decay, gum disease, or both.
   a. Formula of dental disease: Of the two foods that feed the bacteria, sugar is the most cariogenic or acid producing. In gum disease the formula is similar except that toxins are produced that contribute to the removal of the protective layer of the gums, resulting in release of serum that flows out to the bacteria through these open lesions.
   b. Forms of sugar: Liquid: Pop, milk on sugared cereal, jello, ice cream, and any sugar foods that become liquid in the mouth. Solid (high percentage of sugar): Candy, pancake syrup. Sticky, retentive: Pastries, macaroni, rice.
   c. Sugar eaten between meals causes decay: This is a statement, no explanation necessary.
   d. Best time to eat sugar is during and at the end of meals: More saliva is present in the mouth during mealtime. The chewing of hard foods stimulates the production of saliva. The ability of the saliva to contribute to the buffering capacity of the plaque appears to correlate with the amount of decay present.
   Discuss the results of the saliva tests taken on visit 3.
   Deficient flow — Caries rate increases. It can be temporary or permanent. It can be due to emotional or physical causes, drugs such as antihistamines, or excessive consumption of refined carbohydrates.
   Abundant flow — Decrease in caries rate.
   High viscosity — Increase in caries rate. The considered cause is excessive and frequent consumption of refined carbohydrates. Reduced sugar intake may help as treatment.
   Low viscosity — Decrease in caries rate.
   Buffering capacity — Related to the bicarbonate buffer system of the body. Poor buffering capacity is associated with rampant decay. Treatment is to eat more fruits and vegetables as they make alkaline residues.
   Excellent capacity is associated with mouths free of decay.
   e. 30 seconds after eating sugar, acid is formed. Sugar remains in my mouth _____ minutes: This time is determined by the oral glu-

cose clearance test, completed at this visit.

f. If bacterial plaque is organized, decay may take place: The visual aid Tablet Test may be used in this discussion. The statement is read to the patient. If it is not understood the explanation is repeated.

g. Modified Snyder test results _____: If the patient's Snyder test is available, it is shown to him; otherwise he is shown a similar test result. (The modified Snyder tests are incubated for 4 days and then discarded.)

Several test tubes representing varying degrees of acidity produced by the bacteria—negative, 1+, 2+, 3+, 4+—are removed from the incubator. The test is explained to the patient in the following manner:

"The medium in the test tube is a carbohydrate. The bacteria in the saliva that was drooled into the test tube use the medium for food, and it is the waste products from the bacteria, or acid, that turn the medium yellow. This test gives an indication of the number of bacteria present; the more bacteria present, the more acid, the more yellow the color. If the tube is completely blue green the test result is negative. If one-fourth of the tube from the top down is yellow the reaction is considered to be 1+, or a small amount of bacteria present. If half of the tube is yellow the reaction is 2+, or a moderate number of bacteria present. If three-fourths of the tube from the top down is yellow the reaction is 3+, or a large number of bacteria present, and if the entire tube is yellow the rating is 4+, an extremely large number of bacteria present.

"This test does not indicate that decay is present or how much decay will occur in the future. A positive test indicates that the conditions that promote decay are present."

Bring into the discussion the information sheet What Should I Eat? and review briefly. In referring to the list of foods to avoid, bring the 5-Day Food Diary into the discussion. The decay-producing foods are identified in the diary and circled in red. The control therapist circles the cariogenic foods in the first 2 days of the 5-Day Food Diary and the patient circles them for the remaining days. Children circle the foods with the assistance of the control therapist.

By circling days 1 and 2 the control therapist shows the patient what foods to include. The patient, by doing days 3, 4, and 5, is actually taking part in the identification. It provides more meaning to him.

If the patient does not return the 5-Day Food Diary, have him recall what he ate the day before. This will provide some information for discussion. It will give an avenue for praise. Once the patient realizes that he will not be ridiculed he will offer more information about his daily food selection so that the session will prove to be a satisfactory one.

Discuss the list, Hidden Sugar: Carbohydrate Evaluation, and the display of test tubes representing popular foods (Fig. 6-7).

Page 3 Food Pattern:

a. Number of meals I eat a day is determined.

b. Number of snacks I eat a day is recorded. Compare this number with that listed on the nutritional record (Fig. 6-25).

c. My favorite snacks: Again compare with the nutritional record.

d. The main decay-producing foods shown in my five day food diary: The foods that have been circled in red are listed in categories, for example, bread, cereal, soft drinks, pastries, candy.

e. The number of times my teeth were exposed to decay-producing foods during this five day period: This is determined by counting all the red circles.

f. The number of times my teeth were exposed to decay-producing foods between meals during this five day period: Count all the red circles listed between meals and record.

g. The number of times my teeth were exposed to decay-producing foods during and at the end of meals during this five day period: This is determined by counting the red circles listed during the meals.

Slowly explain that during and at the end of the meal are the good times for exposure, whereas between meals is the decay-producing time. Continue by explaining that during this particular week that he was keeping the 5-Day Food Diary he was also flossing and brushing his teeth and the bacteria were not present in an organized mass.

Ask the patient directly if he understands the role that sugar and flour play in the decay process. If he does not, repeat the explanation of the mechanism of disease from the beginning (Chapter 4).

h. Snack food is usually sugar and/or starch containing no vitamins or minerals: These foods satisfy the appetitite to the extent that well-balanced meals are not eaten. The lack of essential vitamins and minerals depletes our bodies, resulting in fatigue, irritability, unhappiness, and ill health.

Allow time for the adult patient to agree with this. A craving for sweets usually indicates a diet low in protein. Increase the protein in order to eliminate the desire for sweets.

Page 4 Why eat food containing vitamins and minerals?

The discussion that follows is in preparation for visit 6 as well as to present a rationale for eating nutritious foods.

a. To control gum disease: Inform the patient of the research of Dr. E. Cheraskin and associates in which it was found that diets high in sucrose and glucose worsen the gingival state, increase the sulcus depth, and tend to increase tooth mobility. Diets high in protein seem to reverse these conditions. It is generally agreed that vitamin C will improve oral conditions in patients with suboptimal blood or tissue level of vitamin C. (Refer to the patient's lingual ascorbic acid test at this time.) Adequate vitamins and minerals along with protein increase the resistance of the patient to disease.

Use demonstration models to point out the gingivae, the sulcus, and the tooth that are dependent on good nutrition.

b. To feel better: All vitamins are necessary but emphasize the vitamin B complex, vitamin E, and vitamin C.

c. To look better: Emphasize vitamin A.

d. Foods to eat between meals: Discuss the picture, Your Snacks: Chance or Choice? As the patient makes positive response to certain foods available to him that he will eat, the food is written down. By this method the patient selects the food that he can and will substitute for the cariogenic ones. The responsibility to follow through is his.

Page 5 My New Habits:

a. The foods I will eat: This is completed as the patient states his intentions.

If rampant decay or a reaction of 4+ on the Snyder test exists, suggest that cariogenic foods be eliminated or that they be limited to two exposures at meals per day for several weeks.

b. The care I give my mouth: This includes the use of floss, brush, and aids specific for the patient.

Page 6 To keep my teeth for lifetime (This is a review of the program to date):

a. *Oral hygiene:* Flossing and brushing the teeth remove the bacteria.

b. *Avoid sugar* and limit white flour to starve the bacteria.

c. *Host resistance* is maintained through optimum nutrition.

d. *The use of fluorides* toughens the teeth. A fluoride toothpaste is suggested.

These comments are written down in the presence of the patient as they are discussed. This allows enough time for the statements being made to be considered and a mental picture to be formed. Ask for questions.

5. Record the patient's oral glucose clearance time and discuss its significance. A high glucose clearance time indicates the patient should avoid sugar foods between meals and maintain a high standard of oral hygiene.

6. Have the patient return to the sink area for the cleaning of the teeth.

7. Have the patient wash his hands.

8. Have the patient be seated.

9. Demonstrate the flossing techniques on the demonstration models. Stress areas and technique needing improvement.

10. Have the patient floss all his teeth, using the floss holder and threader as needed.

11. Have the patient use the Perio-Aid as needed.

12. Have the patient rinse his mouth.

13. Place the chest towel on the patient.

14. Demonstrate the toothbrushing technique on the patient's diagnostic models. Have children demonstrate technique on models. Correct the technique as needed.

15. Have patient brush all his teeth, using the sulcular brush and Proxabrush as needed, clean appliances, and rinse his mouth.

16. Have patient put Vaseline on lips and fingers to prevent staining from the disclosant.

17. Have the patient stain his teeth and appliances and rinse his mouth.

18. The control therapist washes her hands.

19. The patient and the control therapist inspect the teeth and appliances for plaque.

20. Have the patient brush the teeth and tongue to remove excessive color.

21. The control therapist washes her hands.

22. Have the patient use the water irrigator if recommended by the dentist.

23. Remove the chest towel from the patient.

24. Have the patient wash his hands if he desires.

25. Make an appointment for visit 6 in approximately 1 week. Time required will be 1 hour. The discussion will concern the patient's nutritional evaluation.

26. Dismiss the patient.

27. Charting

a. Record areas of plaque (after cleaning), bleeding, and tenderness on Disease Control Check List.

b. Make recommendations for visit 6 on Personal Observation Record.

DISEASE CONTROL
Visit 6

Preparation Before Visit 6

1. Record the results of the nutritional evaluation on the patient's Nutritional Record.

2. Mark in red the nutrients listed below 100 per cent RDA on the computer printout and the Foods High in Essential Nutrients. This is for easy identification by the patient.

3. Draw a line under the Recommended Daily Dietary Allowances that correspond with the patient's age and sex. This is used for an appreciation of the standards as they relate to the patient.

4. Draw lines on the computer printout between the following nutrients:

Vitamin B_1 to niacin and calories

Vitamin B$_6$ to protein
Vitamin E to vitamin A
Pantothenic acid to vitamin C
Calcium to phosphorus
This is used in discussing these nutrients and their relationship to each other.

5. Prepare the Personal Dental Profile (Fig. 6-26).
6. Make additional information sheets ready for the patient.

The Visit

Time allowed for appointment: 60 minutes
Place: The control room
Persons involved: The patient and the control therapist
Short-range goals:
1. To identify any inadequacies that may exist in the diet.
2. To recognize how inadequacies can be corrected.
Long-range goal:
To improve faulty food selection and eating patterns and change them to ones that are conducive to good dental health.
Equipment:
Counter space
  Models of teeth with demonstration brush
  Visuals aids: Food labels and food models as needed
  Take-home packet including:
    Nutritional evaluation (Figs. 6-10, 6-11)
    Recommended Daily Dietary Allowances (Fig. 6-1)
    Foods High in Essential Nutrients (Fig. 6-13)
    Computer printout (Fig. 6-12)
    A Guide to Good Eating (Fig. 6-2)
  Diet Evaluation form with the patient's 5-Day Food Diary (Fig. 6-18).
  Information sheets and pamphlets as needed:
    Meal Planning (Fig. 6-20)
    How to Have a Happy Day (Fig. 6-21)
    To Save Dollars (Fig. 6-22)
    Children (Fig. 6-24)
    Happy Birthday Suggestions (Fig. 6-23)
    Your Food: Chance or Choice?
    How Do You Score on Nutrition? (Fig. 6-4)

Home care prescription week 3 (Fig. 5-56)
Sink counter space
  Two hand towels
  The patient's chest towel and neck clip
  Patient's toothbrush and Proxabrush, Floss threader, irrigator, Floss holder and Perio-Aid as needed
  Patient's toothpaste
  Diagnostic models of the patient's teeth
  Mouth mirror
  Patient's drinking cup
  Disclosing tablet
  Vaseline on 2-by-2-inch gauze
  Dental floss
  Flashlights
Procedure:
1. The control therapist greets the patient.
2. Have the patient wash his hands.
3. Have the patient be seated.
4. Have the patient floss all his teeth using the floss holder and threader as needed. To obtain a true evaluation of the patient's ability to clean his teeth, the flossing and brushing techniques are not demonstrated prior to cleaning at this visit.
5. Have the patient use the Perio-Aid as needed.
6. Have the patient rinse his mouth.
7. Place the chest towel on the patient.
8. Have the patient brush all of his teeth, using the Proxabrush as needed, clean appliances, and rinse his mouth.
9. Review home care prescription week 3 (adults disclose once a month; children disclose once a week).
10. The Plak-Lite is used for disclosing the teeth with the appliances in place. Have the patient rinse his mouth four or five times. The Plak-Lite is used to familiarize the patient with the products that are commercially available.
11. The control therapist washes her hands.
12. The patient and the control therapist inspect the teeth and appliances.
13. If necessary, demonstrate the brushing technique.
14. Have the patient brush his teeth and tongue to remove the excessive color.
15. The control therapist washes her hands.

16. Have the patient use the water irrigator if recommended by the dentist.
17. Remove the chest towel from the patient.
18. Have the patient wash his hands if he desires.
19. Invite the patient to the area designated for further nutritional counseling.

    Since the individual is respected for his intelligence, and the majority are familiar with meal planning and preparation, this discussion is handled as an informative review. Through the discussion of his nutritional analysis, the patient is aware of possible nutrient deficiencies and is motivated to learn how to correct them.

20. Using the Recommended Daily Dietary Allowances, Revised 1968, indicate to the patient the grouping he is in and the amount of nutrients that has been suggested. His requirements may be higher because of his state of health and mental stress. Emphasize that this information provides a guide for diet planning.
21. Using the visual aid display of labels, discuss the minimum daily adult requirement as compared to the recommended daily dietary allowance. Discuss the ingredients as listed on the labels.
22. Review with the patient the nutritional evaluation. As each nutrient or nutrient factor is discussed, the actual amount is compared with the RDA for that patient. Throughout the counseling the patient refers to the Foods High in Essential Nutrients. Nutrients that are less than the 100 per cent RDA have been marked in red for easy patient identification. By referring to this list, the patient realizes his deficiencies because he is not eating the food source.

    After the printout figures have been reviewed, discuss the lines that were drawn on the printout indicating the relationship between nutrients.

    Vitamin B_6 requirements may increase with increased protein intake.
    Vitamin B_1 and niacin needs increase with caloric intake.

Vitamins E and A are necessary to keep the lung tissue healthy.

Pantothenic acid and vitamin C are used by the body in times of stress.

As polyunsaturates are increased the need for vitamin E increases.

Equal amounts of calcium and phosphorus appear to be necessary for effective utilization in the body. Some believe that a phosphorus-to-calcium ratio of 2 to 1, or 0.5, contributes to the prevention of decay. The amount of calcium consumed should be at least the minimum RDA.

The purpose of this discussion is so the patient will realize some of the complexities involved as the vitamins and minerals work together to provide better health.

Occasionally a patient will question the validity of the evaluation. To be sure, it is only as accurate as the patient who completed the form. It is advisable to say as little as possible. Be sympathetic; do not be critical of his accuracy in completing the questionnaire.

Return to the form and briefly check a few foods for errors. Occasionally someone will forget to check eggs; however, experience indicates that patients make fairly accurate accountings. Only the patient knows for sure. This same patient will improve his eating habits and will inform you of this change on his next visit.

Dietronics will indicate inadequacies. Supplements may be prescribed by the dentist on the basis of his diagnosis. The patient is encouraged to improve his food selection and eating habits.

23. The optimum diet is discussed.

    For the patient who does not return the nutritional evaluation questionnaire, continue with planning the optimum diet. This patient will accept and even participate in the discussion.

24. Using a Guide to Good Eating, lead the patient into a discussion of the optimum diet and how to select it. Discuss each

group individually, pointing out specific foods, the nutrients they largely supply, what constitutes a serving, and the minimal recommended number of servings each day. This grouping of food is familiar to most people except perhaps the young child who has not been exposed to it yet in school. The reasons for applying this information have usually been forgotten by the patient.

25. Using the work sheet Diet Evaluation transpose the foods listed in the 5-Day Food Diary into the four food groupings. The control therapist demonstrates to the patient by completing days 1 and 2. The patient completes days 3, 4, and 5. The average is determined and compared with the suggested minimum servings.

    The purpose of this exercise is to have the patient become aware of the types of food he is eating within the basic four food groups and to determine any inadequacies.

    "What I Need" is completed by the patient as he himself suggests the foods he can eat or omit to improve his food selection.

26. Give adults the day-by-day pamphlet from *How Do You Score on Nutrition?* This form is not returned to the office unless the patient has a question and desires more information. Its purpose is to continue the enthusiasm at home that was generated at this visit.

27. Provide the patient with informational sheets that meet his needs. All adults receive Meal Planning, How to Have a Happy Day, and To Save Dollars. Adults with children receive Happy Birthday Suggestions and Children.

28. Review with the patient his Personal Dental Profile. The patient now understands why he may feel as he does. He is aware of nutrients and those that he is deficient in, and he knows the food they represent. He has been reminded or perhaps has learned for the first time how to plan a balanced meal. Not once

in this discussion was he told he should eat more of a certain food. He realized this himself. It is important that the patient be allowed to make his own decisions. The responsibility of the control therapist is to present facts and to supply possible solutions, but unless the patient makes the final decision, it will not be carried through.

29. The next appointment of the control program is in 1 month. Time required will be 30 minutes.

    The patient is now ready for calculus removal, fluoride polish, and fluoride treatment. Have the patient make appointment with the receptionist.

30. Dismiss the patient.

31. Charting
    a. Record areas of plaque (after cleaning), bleeding, and tenderness on Disease Control Check List.
    b. Make recommendations for visit 7 on Personal Observation Record.
    c. Complete the recall record.

Variations in Procedure for Young People, Aged 6 to 17 Years in Visit 6

1. Filmstrips are viewed at the beginning of control visit 6.
   Judy's Family Food Notebook for children 5 to 12 years.
   Vitamins and You for young people 12 to 17 years.

2. Immediately following the filmstrip, the patient plans an adequate breakfast, lunch, and dinner, using the plastic food models (Fig. 6-8) and A Guide to Good Eating. As the young people arrange and rearrange the food, the four food groups are discussed.

3. Complete the worksheet Diet Evaluation (visit 6)

4. Review their nutritional evaluation with them (visit 6).

5. Have the youth measure out the number of teaspoons of sugar that appears in the printout. The sugar is transferred from the sugar jar and placed into an empty

bowl: 48 teaspoons equals 1 cup. The average for the child is about 1 cup.

6. Review labels with the children from grade 5 and up.
7. Provide the teenagers with the pamphlet *Your Food: Chance or Choice?*
8. Have the patient complete the oral hygiene procedures (visit 6).

Applying Control Measures to Children

The age the child goes through the control program is determined by the dentist. A 5-year-old or kindergarten child can usually brush his teeth fairly well. The 6-year-old can usually floss his teeth using an aid. Some 6-year-olds, especially girls, can finger the floss. This depends upon the coordination of the child.

A suggested schedule follows:

Age 2. The mother goes on to the control program and she will in turn floss and brush the child's teeth and should continue until he is about 5 years of age.

Up until the age of 5 years the child has not developed his motor coordination. He does not develop until about the age of 3 years the ability to do both the vertical and the horizontal strokes that are used in the brushing technique. It is not until the age of 5 that he begins to adequately handle the pencil and his eating utensils. Usually the mother is anxious for the child to become independent, and brushing his own teeth is a signal that he is finally beginning to do something for himself. The mother can be told that she should be cleaning Jimmy's teeth, but she will not hear. For this reason the mother must control her own disease. She must realize the importance of what and why she is doing it. Jimmy can and should be encouraged to continue to brush his teeth, but he cannot be responsible for cleaning them. When the mother goes through the control program the educational material is adjusted to include material for the child, and home supplies are provided for both the parent and the child.

Ages 3 through 4. The mother and child go on the control program together. The mother learns the techniques and repeats them on the child.

Age 5. During this period and continuing through the teen years, the child goes on to the control program alone without the presence of a relative.

This is the beginning of the one-to-one relationship that is established in the control program. Mothers usually do not perform well in the presence of children. They are usually too concerned over the children's behavior, and consequently nothing is achieved and the time is wasted.

If children are 5 to 8 years old and the mother has not been through the control program, the mechanism of disease as well as the oral hygiene techniques are discussed separately with the mother so that she will understand the purpose and the methodology.

At age 5, the child will be able to brush his teeth. The mother will have to floss the teeth, using an aid, and will be required to check the child's teeth for the removal of plaque. The child will also begin to learn that sugar foods are harmful and should not be eaten between meals and that there are foods that will make him feel good and grow big.

Age 6 to 7. These children will be able to floss their teeth, using an aid. Some children can finger the floss. The mother needs to check the teeth for plaque, see that the flossing and brushing are done, and occasionally supervise the technique. The child will learn about nutrition as related to health.

Age 8 to 12. These children should learn to finger the floss. There will be exceptions. They can adequately brush their teeth. The mother will need to see that it is done; she will need to check the teeth for plaque and occasionally supervise the techniques. The child will learn about nutrition.

After the child is 8 years old, the mother is not given specific oral hygiene instructions. The mother of a child between 5 and approximately 16 years of age meets with the control therapist about 2 weeks into the program for a complete résumé as well as nutritional counseling applicable to her youngster.

The two major roles the mother plays in preventing decay and bleeding gums are: She must encourage the child to floss and brush, and she must check his technique. She must encourage good eating habits and provide food selections that are conducive to maintaining dental health.

Suggestions for Implementing Control for Children. Stress to the mother that sulcular brushing should be done only once a day. If the mother cleans the child's teeth too often during the day, the child will become tired and uncooperative. Suggest that the child or mother clean the child's teeth after dinner rather than just before bedtime. Both the child and the mother will be more rested.

Important: The mother is always responsible for checking the teeth after the disclosant has been used. This practice should be continued for as many years into the teens as possible.

The Appointment for Mothers of Children Aged 5 Years to Late Teens

1. This visit is for 30 minutes with the mother alone. It is held after the return of the nutritional evaluation (visit 6).
2. Review with the mother the oral hygiene techniques and the reasons for them.
3. Discuss the patient's Preventive Measures for Your Dental Health, nutritional evaluation and Personal Dental Profile with the mother. Provide additional materials and information as needed.
4. Provide a Disease Control Family Summary sheet when more than one member of the family is going through the program.

DISEASE CONTROL
Visit 7

Time allowed for appointment: 30 minutes
Place: The control room
Persons involved: The patient and the control therapist
Goals:
1. To determine the conduciveness of the patient's mouth to decay.

2. To review with the patient the food factors involved in dental disease.
3. To review with the patient the oral hygiene techniques.
4. To motivate the patient to care for himself.

Equipment:
Counter space:
Models of teeth with demonstration brush
Pictures of the oral hygiene techniques, such as those in Chapter 5
Booklets: *A Boy and His Physique; A Girl and Her Figure* (Chapter 6)
Snyder test and 15-minute caries conduciveness test (Chapter 4)
Bag for supplies
Two packets of disclosing wafers
One spool of dental floss
Patient's toothbrush and toothpaste
Sink counter space:
Two hand towels
The patient's chest towel and neck clip
Patient's toothbrush and Proxabrush core, Floss threader, Floss holder, Perio-Aid and water spray as necessary
Patient's toothpaste
Diagnostic models of the patient's teeth
Mouth mirror
Patient's drinking cup
Disclosing tablet
Vaseline on 2-by-2-inch gauze
Dental floss
Flashlights
Procedure:
1. The control therapist greets the patient.
2. Have the patient wash his hands.
3. Have the patient be seated.
4. Place the chest towel on the patient.
5. Have the patient drool saliva into the Snyder test medium. The purpose of this test is to determine the amount of *Lactobacillus acidophilus* in the mouth. It is conducted prior to cleaning the teeth. A letter stating the results is mailed to each patient (Fig. 3-19).
6. Conduct the 15-minute caries conduciveness test. This measures the enzyme, reductase. It is felt that these results are related to the effectiveness of the flossing and brushing techniques. Ex-

perience with this test has shown that even though the Snyder test reaction is 4+ the mouth may still be nonconducive or only slightly conducive to caries production.

7. Discuss with the patient his food selection, eating habits, and food supplementation, and how he generally feels emotionally and physically.

8. Demonstrate on models the flossing technique. Show illustrations of the proper technique. The review is necessary because of the time interval since visit 6.

9. Have the patient floss all his teeth, using the floss holder and threader as needed.

10. Have the patient use the Perio-Aid as needed.

11. Have the patient rinse his mouth.

12. Have the patient put Vaseline on his fingers and lips to prevent staining.

13. Disclose the teeth with Displaque. The blue areas are thick, older areas of plaque and indicate where assistance in the technique is needed.

14. Demonstrate on the models the toothbrushing technique. Have the child demonstrate the technique on the models. Show illustrations of the proper technique.

15. Have the patient brush all his teeth, using the Proxabrush as needed, and clean appliances.

16. The control therapist washes her hands.

17. The patient and the control therapist inspect the teeth and appliances for plaque.

18. Have the patient brush his teeth and tongue to remove excessive color.

19. The control therapist washes her hands.

20. Have the patient use the water irrigator if recommended by the dentist.

21. Remove the chest towel from the patient.

22. Have the patient wash his hands if he desires.

23. The teenage boy is given the pamphlet *A Boy and His Physique*, and the teenage girl is given *A Girl and Her Figure*.

24. The patient is placed on the recall list for visit 8. His supplies, including the toothbrush he has been using from visit 1 to visit 7, are given to him.

25. Dismiss the patient.

26. Charting
    a. Disease Control Check List
    b. Personal Observation Record
    c. Recall File
    d. Test Records

DISEASE CONTROL
Visit 8

Time allowed for appointment: 30 minutes
Place: The control room
Persons involved: The patient and the control therapist
Goals:

1. To determine the conduciveness of the patient's mouth to decay.

2. To review with the patient the oral hygiene techniques.

3. To review with the patient the food factors involved in dental disease.

4. To motivate the patient to care for himself.

Equipment:
Counter space:
  Models of teeth with demonstration brush
  Snyder test and 15-minute caries test
  Bag for supplies
    2 packets of disclosing tablets
    1 spool of dental floss
    Patient's toothbrush and toothpaste
  Preventive recall card completed—schedule of appointments (Fig. 3-11)
  Patient's preventive recall card—the visit for the dentist for about 1 year after the previous prophylaxis
Sink counter space:
  Two hand towels
  The patient's chest towel and neck clip
  New toothbrush and Proxabrush core, Floss holder, Floss threader, Perio-Aid and water spray as needed
  New toothpaste
  Diagnostic models of the patient's teeth
  Mouth mirror
  Patient's drinking cup
  Disclosing tablet
  Vaseline on 2-by-2-inch gauze
  Dental floss
  Flashlights

Procedure:

1. The control therapist greets the patient.
2. Have the patient wash his hands.
3. Have the patient be seated.
4. Have the patient drool saliva into the Snyder test medium.
5. Conduct the 15-minute caries test.
6. Demonstrate on the models the flossing technique.
7. Have the patient floss all his teeth, using the floss holder and threader as needed.
8. Have the patient use the Perio-Aid as needed. Have the patient rinse his mouth.
9. Have the patient place Vaseline on his lips and fingers.
10. Have the patient disclose his teeth with Dis-plaque with appliances in place.
11. Demonstrate on the models the tooth-brushing technique. Have the child demonstrate the technique on models.
12. Have the patient brush all his teeth, using a Proxabrush as needed, and clean the appliances.
13. The control therapist washes her hands.
14. The patient and the control therapist inspect the teeth and appliances for plaque.
15. Have the patient brush his teeth and tongue to remove color.
16. The control therapist washes her hands.
17. Have the patient use the water irrigator if recommended by the dentist.
18. Remove the chest towel from the patient.
19. Have the patient wash his hands if he desires.
20. Ascertain the frequency of flossing, brushing, staining, and the use of water spray.
21. Review with the patient the conditions that exist in his mouth.
22. Discuss food selection.
23. Inform the patient of the recall procedure. Patients are seen once a year by the control therapist and dentist. Time interval between each visit is 6 months.
24. Give the patient his supplies.
25. Dismiss the patient.
26. Charting
    a. Disease Control Check List
    b. A Disease Control Program Completion Letter (Fig. 3-20) containing the result of the Snyder test is mailed in approximately 7 days.

CONCLUSIONS

Each individual requires a personalized approach. Everyone is unique as a person confronted with different problems that dictate solutions that are applicable to him alone. An outline of a comprehensive program for the control of dental disease may be all-inclusive except that it does not take into account the variables or describe patient's need, personalities, interests, and past experiences that make each patient special. What has been presented is the basic approach and knowledge that form the keystone of a control program. Common sense, logic, and a feeling towards others are what contribute to communication between people.

Preventive Maintenance

THE VIEW FOLLOWING DISEASE CONTROL

When the dentist again enters into the picture to care for the patient, changes have taken place within the patient's mouth. There is a marked contrast in the oral conditions of those who have been through a disease control program, such as the one described in Chapter 8, and those who have not. It was general experience before disease control that attractive people would present themselves with heavy calculus and plaque and exhibit profuse bleeding when the teeth were cleaned. The hemorrhaging was so enormous, in many instances, that it was very difficult to see the gingivae and the sulcus of the teeth. After having experienced the changes that take place, one cannot continue in the ways of the past. To practice without disease control is futile and a continuation of ignorance that is without justification or good common sense.

THE CHANGE

The disease control program has made a believer of the patient. This has come about through change in the feel of his mouth. It is when he next sees the dentist that the patient wants and must have the reassurance and praise for the progress that he has made. It is with much satisfaction that this observation can be made. Not only have clinical changes taken place, but also the attitude has changed, which creates a person who is more confident and prepared for dental procedures that will correct, restore, and replace that which has been effected by dental disease. The patient is more relaxed and accepting of the dental treatment that lies ahead. A more normal relationship exists between the dentist and the patient. The fear and uncertainity of dentistry have been greatly reduced.

Clinically, the procedures of removing calculus and polishing the teeth are greatly simplified. Less time is required. Bleeding is minimal or nonexistent and with little discomfort experienced by the patient. The placement of the rubber dam is less traumatic to the patient because he has become accustomed to the use and feel of dental floss in his mouth. The gum tissue is healthy, and there is not the discomfort and bleeding that previouly were associated with the application of floss. In contrast, the patient who does not floss is resentful and bothered by the introduction of devices or manipulation of the oral tissues. This point is magnified with children. The difference is quite dramatic.

Certainly, better treatment can be accomplished by having the gingival tissue in a healthy condition. This will be reflected in better marginal integrity of castings or restorative materials, not to mention the

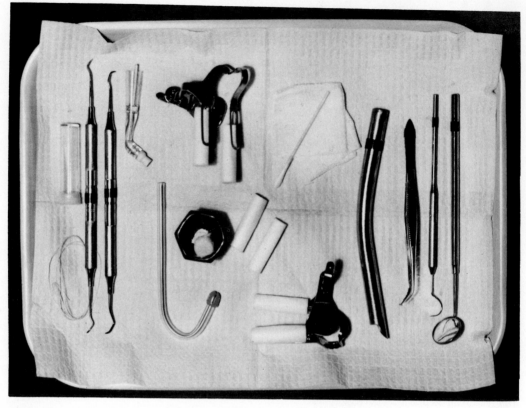

FIG. 9-1. The fluoride treatment tray.

saving of emotional wear and tear on the dentist in trying to maintain a dry field.

It becomes very difficult for a dentist, once he has been exposed to patients with their disease under control, to treat patients who have not received the benefits of the program. Emergency treatment is provided willingly and with empathy, but continuing on into a treatment situation with bacterial infection provides little satisfaction, as compared to first promoting health.

TOPICAL APPLICATION OF FLUORIDE

As a part of the preventive procedure in this text, stannous fluoride treatment is given to all children and adults following visit 6 of the disease control program. For the adult, the fluoride treatment is repeated yearly for three times and continued thereafter if the decision is made that additional treatments might be of value to the patient. For children, fluoride is applied every 6 months for three times, and application is repeated as new teeth erupt.

If fluoride is not in the water supply, it is suggested that it be given as drops. The total dosage should be divided and consumed throughout the day. It is preferred that it be taken in water or fruit juice, not milk, as the calcium in milk interferes with the absorption of the fluoride.

Procedure:

One drop of 8 per cent stannous fluoride is added to the stannous fluoride paste, and the teeth are polished after the calculus has been removed. The teeth are flossed. A topical application of stannous fluoride solution is made to the surface of the teeth and allowed to remain 30 seconds.

Tray Setup (Fig. 9-1):

Mirror

Explorer

Cotton pliers

Vacu-tip

Saliva ejector

Dampen dish with Zircate treatment paste to which has been added one drop of fluoride solution

Disposable prophy angle with rubber cup

Straight perio instrument

Contrangle (double ended) perio instrument

6 cotton rolls

2-by-2-inch gauze

Cotton applicator

Dental floss

1 vial 8 per cent stannous fluoride crystals 0.4 gm.

Distilled water

Left and right Garmer's clamps

Method:

1. Prepare a fresh 8 per cent stannous fluoride solution by placing distilled water within ¼ inch from the top in the vial

PREVENTIVE MAINTENANCE RECORD

Name _____ Chart # _____ Disease Control

Yes
No
Need

Date					
Tests					
Snyder Test					
Vitamin C Test					
Tongue					
State of health					
Cleanliness					
Color					
Gingivae Appearance					
Health					
Reduction of edema					
Inflammation reduction					
Bleeding reduction					
Areas of bleeding					
Cheeks					
Normal appearance					
Color					
Lips					
Color					
Moist or dry					
Crusting					
Enlargement					
Ulceration					
Angular fissuring					
Scarring					
Teeth					
Disclosant					
Plaque Index past staining					
Appearance of teeth					
Calculus Formation Index					
Mobility					
Caries Evaluation					
Complaint Improvement					
Sensitive teeth					
Sore mouth					
Pain					
Tenderness					
Dry mouth, excessive saliva					
X-ray Examination					
Prophylaxis					
Fluoride Treatment					
Improvement points					

FIG. 9-2. Preventive Maintenance Record.

provided by the manufacturer. Replace cap. Shake well until mixed. (The stannous fluoride solution is not clear because of hydrolysis.) The solution retains its effectiveness for only 30 to 45 minutes.

2. Scale each tooth of calculus.
3. Polish each tooth at slow speed for approximately 10 seconds with Zircate treatment paste to which has been added 1 drop of free stannous fluoride. Use unwaxed dental floss to draw excess Zircate paste through the interproximal areas. Have the patient rinse the material from his mouth.
4. Isolate one lower quadrant with a Garmer's clamp and the upper quadrant with a cotton roll between the cheek and the teeth. The cotton rolls should be completely clear of the tooth surface so that the applied stannous fluoride is not absorbed. Dry the teeth.
5. Apply stannous fluoride solution to the surface of the teeth with a cotton-tipped applicator; keep the teeth moist with the solution for 30 seconds.
6. Repeat the steps taken on the opposite side.
7. Allow the patient to rinse his mouth.

PREVENTIVE MAINTENANCE RECALL

This is the recall visit with the dentist for all patients.

Time allowed for appointment: 30 minutes
Tray setup:
  Fluoride treatment tray
  Cavitron instrument
  Modified Snyder test
  Lingual ascorbic acid test
  Stopwatch
Procedure:
1. The health history is updated.
2. The chair-side assistant escorts the patient to the operatory, places the chest towel on the patient, and indicates to the dentist that the patient is ready (Valcom signal system).
3. Dentist enters and greets the patient.
4. The Preventive Maintenance Record (Fig. 9-2) is completed.

5. The modified Snyder test is taken.
6. The lingual ascorbic acid test is taken.
7. The necessary x-rays are taken.
8. If the patient's disease is not under control, the statement is made by the dentist that research has found that decay and periodontal disease are infections. This can lead to the viewing of the plaque under the microscope and the development of the patient's desire to proceed into the control of his disease through a control program. The prophylaxis, fluoride application, and needed treatment would follow after the patient has controlled his disease.
9. If the patient has his disease under control, the preventive philosophy and preventive measures are discussed. The prophylaxis and fluoride treatment are given. The patient is rescheduled in the recall file.
10. If the patient has been through the control program and continues to display disease, he is scheduled for preventive recall visits as determined by the dentist.

DISEASE CONTROL RECALL

Time allowed for appointment: 30 minutes
Place: The control room
Persons involved: The patient and the control therapist
Goals:
1. To assist the patient in the oral hygiene techniques.
2. To discuss and encourage food selections and eating habits that are conducive to *good health.*
3. To conduct tests to determine the conduciveness of the mouth to dental disease.
4. To motivate the patient to continued action.
Equipment:
Counter space:
  Models of teeth with demonstration toothbrush
  Snyder test agar, 15-minute caries conduciveness test
  Plastic bag for supplies
    one spool of unwaxed dental floss
    two packets of disclosing tablets

Recall appointment card listing the month of the next visit (Chapter 3)

Sink counter space:

Two hand towels

Chest towel and neck clip

New toothbrush and Proxabrush core, Floss holder, Floss threader, Perio-Aid and water spray as needed.

New toothpaste

Mouth mirror

Patient's drinking cup

Disclosing tablet

Vaseline on 2-by-2-inch gauze

Dental floss

Flashlight

Procedure:

1. The patient is greeted by the control therapist.
2. The patient completes the form, Disease Control Recall—Food Habits (Fig. 9-3).
3. The procedure is the same as outlined for visit 8 of the control program, (Chapter 8). The check list (Fig. 9-4) is used for charting, with each section representing a separate control visit.

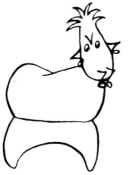

DISEASE CONTROL RECALL

Food Habits

Name _____

Date _____

1. Please list what you ate yesterday.
   Breakfast:

   Snacks:

   Lunch

   Snacks:

   Dinner:

2. What did you eat last night before you went to bed?

3. Did you eat breakfast this morning?

4. What beverages have you been drinking?

   Milk   Kool-Aid

   Pop   Fruit juices

   Hot chocolate   Others - list

FIG. 9-3. Disease Control Recall—Food Habits.

EVALUATING THE RESULTS

It is of value to know the effectiveness of a disease control program on the behavioral changes and the control achieved over dental disease. In order to obtain this information and to command an overall view of the results of dental education, it is necessary to evaluate each patient at subsequent recall visits. This evaluation serves to inform the dental staff of the progress that has been made or to point out deficiencies or goals that are left unattained. Whether it is negative or positive input, the determination helps to guide the dental educator in implementing a successful program.

Passage of time is required to allow a comparison between the conditions that existed before and the change that has occurred to provide the current status of health of the individual. For the patient, the

DISEASE CONTROL RECALL

Name _____   Chart # _____

Date						
Fifteen Minute Caries Test						
Snyder Test						
Frequency of Flossing						
Frequency of Brushing						
Frequency of Staining						
Use of special tools, Proxabrush, Perio-Aid						
Use of Water Spray						
Oral Hygiene Index past staining						
Discussion of foods						
Use of food supplements						
Recall						
Home supplies						
Comments						

FIG. 9-4. Disease Control Recall—an evaluation form.

short-term evaluation or awareness is most important for he can feel and taste the difference, and he has gained assurance that his mouth smells better and that his teeth are more attractive. The long-term evaluation becomes important to him because it tells him that he is still on the right track, and there is definite evidence of the effort that he is expending. The reinforcement that he receives further helps to motivate his action.

COLLECTING THE APPROPRIATE DATA

The basic steps in the evaluation of the preventive program are to determine what criteria are needed and the method of obtaining the information. Data are collected on charts or check lists or both. The tabulation of data provides a means of formulating conclusions.

The continuing interest of the control staff is dependent upon the results of the control program and how the test results correlate with clinical symptoms. The collection of data should be started with the very first patient who enters into a control program. It may require several minutes to tabulate the test results, but it is a monumental task at a later date to sift back through charts to obtain information.

The long-term goals can be evaluated at the time of the patient's recall by following the Preventive Maintenance Record (Fig. 9-2). This serves as both a means of recording information and a check list to be followed in the procedure for the recall appointment. Through discussion, observation, and completion of this quality control form, information is gathered. The patient is directly and indirectly informed through this method of his progress. He should be aware of it himself, but he appreciates its recognition by the dentist.

Other methods of filing information are by tabulation on cards and the use of notebooks. The design of the data-collecting sheets and filing system will depend upon the information that the dentist wishes to obtain.

CONCLUSIONS

It takes only one case to determine that the path of prevention is the right one. Each case after the first reinforces the fact that it can be accomplished readily and that control is obtainable. The variations that make preventive dentistry interesting are provided by the patient with his individual needs and differences. Success is achieved through answering the questions that are created in the patient's mind. It has been an educational experience that directly relates to him. In each and every instance, an improvement has been noted. The choices that he will make in the brushing of his teeth, in the foods he will eat, and in the selection of his toothpaste, dental floss, and toothbrush will be based upon knowledge rather than chance or indecision.

In our control program, the patient is not asked to evaluate the program. The patient is being treated for his disease. It is questionable if the patient really knows if the program is good. He really knows only what it did for him now. The long-range results will take years to evaluate. The dental staff will know what the program has done for the patient because it did the same for them.

LOOKING TOWARD CHANGE

Periodontal disease is tied closely to bacteria, but what other factors are involved? What is the role of the bacterial enzymes and endotoxins? Is it an immune response or an antigen-antibody reaction? What is the mechanism whereby the white blood cells can destroy tissue as an aftermath of fighting infections? In dental decay, are further answers needed concerning the role of the calcium : phosphorus ratio? What is the significance of the voltage created by the bacterial plaque? Is the role of sugar significant in changing the fluid-transfer mechanism inside the tooth to create a cause-and-effect relationship that makes teeth more susceptible to decay?

It is more than likely that there are factors involved in dental disease other than those implicated in the acid-decay theory and more complex than just the toxic effects of bacteria upon periodontal tissues. What is wanted is a method of application that works now, but in our haste we must carefully sort what is true from what we wish were true. In contrast, an attempt has to be made not to hold too firmly to the old comfortable beliefs at the expense of rejecting other factors that are relevant. What was held to be true yesterday may not be necessarily true today. Each dentist is, in a sense, a researcher observing, studying, and considering new concepts.

Testing is not done entirely in a laboratory. We are living in a laboratory called life. As you develop the preventive practice, think of the woodsman philosopher who said, "You no more can teach what you ain't learned than come from some place you ain't been."

Bibliography

Abrahamson, E. M., and Pezet, A. W.: Body, Mind and Sugar. New York, Holt, 1951.

Amenta, C. A., and Brackett, R. C.: Dialogue on Preventive Dentistry. Chicago, March Pub. Co. 1972.

Arnim, S.: Dental irrigation—its place in the total concept of oral hygiene. Dent. Pract. 3:7-10, 1965.

Barkley, R. F.: Toothbrushing—the hoax of American dentistry. Ariz. Dent. J., 13:14-16 (15 Nov.) 1967.

——: How to find and keep the rare gem. Dent. Manag., 12:53-66 passim (July) 1972.

——: Successful Preventive Dental Practice. Macomb, Ill., Preventive Dentistry Press, 1972.

Berland, T. and Seyler, A. E.: Your Children's Teeth; A Complete Guide for Parents. New York, Meredith, 1968.

Berne, E.: Games People Play. New York, Grove, 1964.

Block, P., Lobene, R. R., and Derdivanis, J. P.: A two-tone dye test for dental plaque. J. Periodontol; 43:423-426 (July) 1972.

Clark, J., W., Cheraskin, E., and Ringsdorf, W. M.: Diet and the Periodontal Patient. Springfield, Ill., Thomas, 1970.

Cohen, D. W., Stoller, N. H., Chace, R., Jr., et al.: A comparison of bacterial plaque disclosants in periodontal disease. J. Periodontol. 43: 333-338 (June) 1972.

Conserving the Nutritive Values in Foods. Washington, Consumer and Food Economics Research Division, Agriculture Research Service, 1971.

Corn, H. and Marks, M. H.: The role of the dental assistant in oral hygiene instruction. Dent. Assist., 38:12-18, (Oct.) 1969.

Craig, G. G. and Dunn, G. R.: A Guide to the Practice of Preventive Dentistry. Sydney, Univ. Sydney, 1971.

Davis, A.: Let's Eat Right to Keep Fit. New York, Harcourt Brace Jovanovich, 1970.

DiOrio, L. P.: A Personalized Program; Educating the Patient in the Prevention of Dental Disease. Chicago, March Pub. Co., 1973.

Dunkin, R. T.: Oral irrigation in your patient's home care control program. J. Amer. Soc. Prevent. Dent. 2:46-47 passim (Mar.-Apr.) 1972.

Eat to Live. Chicago, Wheat Flour Institute, 1970.

Fast, J.: Body Language. New York, M. Evans and Co., 1970.

Fitch, M., and Moxley, R.: Preventive dentistry with behavior modification. J. Amer. Soc. Prevent. Dent., 2:45-46 (Sept.-Oct.) 1972.

Fleishman, A.: Sense and Nonsense. San Francisco, International Society for General Semantics, 1971.

Food Before Six—A Feeding Guide for Parents of Young Children. Chicago, National Dairy Council, 1968.

Ginott, H. G.: Between Parent and Child. New York, Avon, 1969.

Given, M.: Modern Encyclopedia of Cooking. pp. 115-119. Chicago, J. G. Ferguson, 1955.

Grant, D., Stern, J. B., and Everett, F. G. (eds.): Orban's Periodontics; A Concept—Theory and Practice. ed. 3. St. Louis, Mosby, 1968.

Groppe, C. C.: A Nutrition Primer. Univ. Calif. Agricultural Extension, HXT-97, 5/71.

——: Meal Planning Patterns, Univ. Calif., Agricultural Extension, HXT-98, 5/71.

A Guide to Good Eating . . . What it Means . . . How to Use It. ed. 2. Chicago, National Dairy Council, 1970.

Indications of nature of food relationships in caries. J. Dent. Res., 49 (suppl.): 1191-1352 (Nov.-Dec.) 1970.

International Conference on Dental Plaque, New York, 1969, presented by the American Dental Association and Warner-Lambert Pharmaceutical Co., Oct. 8, 1969. Morris Plains, N. J., Warner-Lambert Pharmaceutical Co., 1970.

Lainson, P. A., Bergquist, J. J., and Fraleigh, C. M.: A Clinical Evaluation of Pulsar, a New Pulsating Water Pressure Cleansing Device. J. Periodontol. 41:401-405 (July) 1970.

Kuhn, B. L.: Dear Juli — Your role in controlling dental disease. Dent. Manag., 11:51-71 passim (June) 1971.

Lang, N. P., Ostergaard, E. and Löe, H.: A fluorescent plaque disclosing agent. J. Periodont. Res., 7:59-67, 1972.

Liljestrand, W. E.: An Engineering Analysis of Oral Irrigators with Respect to their Washing Ability. Texell Products Co., Houston, Tex.

Maltz, M.: Psycho-Cybernetics. North Hollywood, Calif. Wilshire Book Co., 1970.

McEnery, E. T., and Suydam, M. J.: Feeding Little Folks. Chicago, National Dairy Council, 1952.

Mittelman, J. S.: Prevention in Dentistry; How We Do It. New York, published by the author, 1969.

Montgomery, A.: The contribution of a dental hygienist to an effective preventive dental practice. J. Amer. Soc. Prevent. Dent., 2:40-41 (Jan.-Feb.) 1972.

National Institute of Dental Research: Research Explores Nutrition and Dental Health. Bethesda, Md. National Institutes of Health, 1970.

———: Research Explores Plaque. Bethesda, Md., National Institutes of Health, 1969.

National Research Council—Food and Nutrition Board: Recommended Dietary Allowances. 7th rev. ed. Washington, National Academy of Sciences—National Research Council, 1968.

Nizel, A. E.: The Science of Nutrition and Its Application in Clinical Dentistry. ed. 2. Philadelphia, Saunders, 1966.

———: Nutrition in Preventive Dentistry: Science and Practice. Philadelphia, Saunders, 1972.

Peshek, R. J.: A Practice Management Manual: A Look Into Practice Management, Emphasis the Super Dentist. 7759 California Ave., Riverside, Calif. 92504, 1970.

Preventive Dentistry. Cincinnati, Ohio, Procter and Gamble Co., 1972.

Rapp, G. W.: A fifteen minute caries test. Ill. Dent. J., 31:290-295 (May) 1962.

Reed, O.: A place for prevention. Dent. Manag., 11:95-96 (June) 1971.

Rehberg, R. E.: How to pick (and train) a preventive assistant. Dent. Eco., 62:36-38 (June) 1972.

Ringsdorf, W., Jr., and Cheraskin, E.: A rapid and simple lingual ascorbic acid test. GP, 25:106-108 (June) 1962.

Schwarzrock, L. H., Schwarzrock, S. P.: Effective Dental Assisting. ed. 2., Dubuque, Iowa, Wm. C. Brown Co., 1959.

Shaner, E. O.: Dental Assistant Rapid Training Manual. Bethesda, Md. 20014 (May) 1972.

Sims, W.: The interpretation and use of the Snyder test and lactobacillus counts. J. Amer. Dent. Ass., 80:1315-1319 (June) 1970.

Stanton, G.: Diet and dental caries, the phosphate sequestration hypothesis, New York Dent. J., 35:399-407 (Aug.-Sept.) 1969.

Steinman, R. R., and Leonora, J.: Relationship of fluid transport through the dentin to the incidence of dental caries. J. Dent. Res., 50:1536-1543 (Nov.-Dec.) 1971.

Weiss, R. L., and Swearingen, R. V.: Chairside Psychology in Patient Education; A Self-Instruction Course. Washington, U. S. Dept. Public Health Service, Division of Dental Health, 1969.

The youngest profession (roundtable discussion). Dent. Manag., 12:20-35 passim (July) 1972.

Zaki, H. A., assisted by Carl L. Bandt, Lars Folke: Clean Teeth Brighten Your Smile! University of Minnesota, 1971.

Index